First Aid for Boaters

First Aid for Boaters

by Alfred W. Kornbluth,
M.D., F.A.C.P.

CROWN PUBLISHERS, INC.   NEW YORK

© 1979 by Alfred W. Kornbluth, M.D.

All rights reserved. No part of this book may be reproduced or utilized in any form or by any means, electronic or mechanical, including photocopying, recording, or by any information storage and retrieval system, without permission in writing from the publisher.
Inquiries should be addressed to Crown Publishers, Inc., One Park Avenue, New York, N.Y. 10016

Printed in the United States of America
Published simultaneously in Canada by
General Publishing Company Limited

Library of Congress Cataloging in Publication Data

Kornbluth, Alfred W
First aid for boaters.

Includes index.
1. First aid in illness and injury.   2. Boats and boating—Accidents and injuries.   I. Title.
[RC88.9.B6K67   1979]   614.8'64   78-26285
ISBN 0-517-53720-6
ISBN 0-517-53721-4 pbk.

To Jean,
who has lovingly filled my life
with comfort and joy,
and to our great kids,
Ronnie, Rick, Donna, and her husband, Ira,
who have embellished that life with laughs, tears, and
love, and have provided a sense of great pride,
this book is sincerely dedicated.

Contents

Preface xi
Introduction 1

1. CRISIS, RESCUE, AND TREATMENT 4
   A Crisis Situation 5
      Rescue 5
      Equipment 5
      When Victim Is Unconscious 8
      Bleeding 14
      Shock 14

2. THE SKIN 17
   Wounds 18
      Abrasions 18
      Avulsion 19
      Incisions and Lacerations 20
      Puncture Wounds 23
      Bee Sting Allergic Reactions 24
      Venomous Snakebites and Poisonous Insects 24
      Injuries by Marine Life 26
      Fishhook Caught in Skin 27
   Boils and Abscesses 28
   Burns 30
   Frostbite 34

3. HEAD INJURIES 35
   Head 35
      Head Injury: Victim Is Conscious 35
      Head Injury: Victim Is Unconscious 37
   Eyes 38
      Foreign Body in the Eye 38
      Pinkeye or Conjunctivitis 38
      Black Eye or Bruise 39
      Snow or Sun Blindness 40

Ears 40
    Earache 40
    Sudden Decrease in Hearing 41
    Dizziness 41
Nose 42
    Nosebleed 42
    Broken Nose 42
    Stuffy or Blocked Nose 43
Mouth 43
    Chapped and Sunburned Lips 43
    Dental Problems 44
    Sore Throat 44
    Obstructed Breathing 45

4. BREATHING AND HEARTBEAT 47
Allergies 47
    Asthma 47
    Injection Procedure 49
    Anaphylactic Shock 51
Chest Injuries 51
    Fractured Ribs 51
    Penetrating Chest Wound 52
Hyperventilation 53
Carbon Monoxide Poisoning 54
Pleurisy-Pneumonia 54
Heart Injury 55
    Angina Pectoris 55
    Heart Attack 56
    Cardiac Arrest 57
    Heart Failure 60
Drowning 61

5. THE GASTROINTESTINAL TRACT 62
Poisoning 62
    Poisoning by Toxic Material 62
    Poisoning by Contaminated Food 64
    Poisoning by Ingestion of Toxic Fish 65
Digestive Disorders 65
    Indigestion 65

Peptic Ulcers 66
Gastroenteritis 67
Constipation 68
Diarrhea 69

Acute Abdominal Pain 69
Mittelschmerz 70
Appendicitis 71
Acute Gallbladder Disease 71
Acute Pancreatitis 72
Kidney Stone 72
Acute Muscle Strain 73
Gas Pocket 73
Ruptured Peptic Ulcer 74

6. THE GENITOURINARY SYSTEM 76
Problems of the Urinary System 76
Urinary Retention 76
Bladder Infection 77
Kidney Stones 78
Problems of the Reproductive System 78
Excessive Vaginal Bleeding 78
Injury or Infection of the Contents of the Scrotum 78

7. MUSCULOSKELETAL INJURIES 79
Muscle Injury 80
Joint Sprains 80
Dislocations 81
Fractures 81
General Measures 81
Closed (Simple) Fractures 83
Open Fracture 88

8. GENERAL BODY DISORDERS 90
Seasickness 91
Hangovers 92
Exposure 93
Heat Exhaustion 93
Heat Stroke 94
Environmental Exposure 95

x   FIRST AID FOR BOATERS

    Unconsciousness   95
        Fainting   95
        Unconsciousness with Convulsions   97
        Faintness and Unconsciousness   98
        Progressive Confusion and Lethargy or Drowsiness   99
        Diabetes   99
        Insulin Reaction   100

9. WATER SAFETY   102
    Be Prepared   102
    Drowning   104
        Immediate Steps   104
        After Six to Twelve Hours   104

10. YOUR FIRST-AID KIT   106
    For Infections with Fever   107
        Antibiotics   107
    For Allergies   108
        Antiallergy Drugs   108
    For Asthma   108
    For Digestive Disorders   108
        Constipation   108
        Diarrhea   109
        Indigestion   109
    For Respiratory Ailments   109
        Cough Suppressants   109
        Nasal or Sinus Blockage   110
    For Pain   110
        Analgesics   110
        Chest Pains   110
    For Seasickness   111
    For Stings   111
    For Sunburn   111
    For Sunscreen   111
    For Acute Anxiety and Insomnia   111
    Miscellaneous   111

Index   113

Preface

In expressing my appreciation to my many friends who have helped in producing this book, it might be best to begin at the beginning, when the idea for writing it was conceived. A friend, medical colleague, fine sailor, and gentleman, Ronald Kaplan, M.D., invited me to present an evening of instruction on emergency medicine to a meeting of the Association of Santa Monica Bay Yacht Clubs. The audience was so hungry for information, and I was so fascinated with the challenge of the material, that it proved to be a most memorable evening. Many others followed.

A review of the literature led to a simplified, explicit summary of the most pertinent information.

The writings and rewritings, typings and retypings, made me increasingly aware of the patience and skill of my secretary-typist, Mrs. Helen Throop, to whom I am most grateful.

The illustrations are the work of Ms. Nina Shapley, one of our students at the University of Southern California Medical School, who managed to sandwich in these artistic efforts between her studies and duties at the Medical Center. Her fine efforts are sincerely appreciated.

Being an internist, I felt the need of an adviser-critic in the form of a surgeon, and I asked Norman Koenig, M.D., for help. Skilled in surgery, experienced especially in burn care, and armed with an extremely literate pen, he whipped sharp edges off the manuscript, keeping my efforts well within the confines of good surgical advice and technique. For his efforts I am extremely grateful.

To Dr. Bernard Becker, an eminent orthopedist, I am indebted for an incisive review and critique of the section in chapter 7 on "those dry bones." His recommendations are always invaluable.

Robert Osterman, M.D., L.L.D., reviewed the book with the eagle eye of a fine surgeon and attorney, and his advice and counsel are most appreciated.

A special note of appreciation goes to Ron Eaton, former publisher of Brooke House, for his confidence in this book, and to Brandt Aymar, Special Projects Editor of Crown Publishers, Inc., for finally delivering this brainchild into the world.

My vote for the most talented, patient, and persevering editors goes to Ruth Glushanok, Barbara Monahan, Auriel Douglas, and Linda Rageh, and with it my sincere thanks.

Having been protected from the world of book publishing, I was not only in dire need of, but also overwhelmed by the advice, enthusiasm, and ideas of Ira Ritter, magazine publisher, and his wife Donna, who also happens to be my daughter. Together they form a brain trust that bears a great responsibility for whatever success this book may enjoy.

Hardly last or least, my friends, Drs. Mae and Jay Ziskin, have earned a special vote of thanks for exposing me to the joy and pain of being an author—and how gratifying and satisfying even that pain can be! To them I will be forever grateful for sharing both the pain and the pleasure.

Introduction

The Next Best Thing to a Doctor Aboard

The sun is shining brightly with a twelve- to fifteen-knot breeze blowing steadily off the starboard beam. The waves are lapping against the hull and the wind whistles softly through the shrouds and trails off the sails' edges. There is a feeling of exhilaration and freedom as all aboard our sailing boat sense the excitement of testing their skills and nautical knowledge against the elements and the unpredictability of nature.

Suddenly there is a thud and a groan and the foredeck "gorilla" falls to the deck holding his leg with an obviously deformed ankle. . . . Or, from the galley comes a scream as your mate accidentally spills a pot of boiling coffee down the side of her thigh. . . . Or, an unexpected jibe; the boom swings—a crack—and your crewman lies unconscious with blood oozing from the side of his forehead.

All those who push off from a dock to go to sea know that the peace and tranquillity of one moment can become pure havoc instants later. That sickening sensation of "Oh, God! What shall I do now?" crops up when most unexpected.

Apparently, many sailors have shared this feeling, because I have been asked as a physician to lecture on first aid to various fleet and yacht clubs

In particular, I have frequently been asked what should be in the first-aid kit aboard an off-shore boat.

While researching this book I became aware of the numerous books that are addressed to the matter of survival, with descriptions of medical or paramedical procedures including emergency appendectomies and intravenous fluid administration on transoceanic ships or top-of-the-world mountain expeditions.

However, little has been available in the way of a *quick* reference handbook for the kinds of urgent situations that often arise in off-shore boating; I mean that ready information about what first aid should be applied during the few hours, or perhaps even a day, that may pass before professional help can be reached.

This book is therefore directed to all those racing enthusiasts, day cruisers, and off-shore skippers who feel a little uneasy at not having a doctor aboard for those unpredictable accidents that can panic and otherwise destroy a beautiful day wherever you may be.

For those planning long trips across water where medical aid will not be accessible for days and where not only first aid but subsequent management would be necessary for prolonged periods of time, there are numerous books and manuals that go more deeply into the procedures to be followed.

For the rest of you who would like to holler "Is there a doctor aboard?" I hope this handbook will serve as the next best thing.

The general format of this book follows what is most apt to happen for the most common injuries. After some initial pearls in chapter 1 on dealing with crises, we go on to discuss the skin in chapter 2. Then we look at the head on your shoulders and proceed down through the body in rather systematic fashion, discussing problems that may arise in each of the body's several systems.

We will end up with a discussion of some of the general illnesses or injuries involving more than one system or part of the body that might befall the person at sea.

The outline of the suggested contents for your first-aid kit can easily be located. It must be emphasized that the contents of this first-aid kit may, of course, change with the advent of new drugs and new methods of management of first-aid problems. By all means, check over this list with your personal physician for prescriptions and for those general items that he agrees you should have aboard. Make sure to check for any allergies or idiosyncrasies to these medicines that you may have.

Certainly individual doctors may differ in their preference for drugs or methods of treatment. There usually is more than one way to manage any medical problem and no promises or guarantees of results are possible.

Follow directions carefully and by all means, if response is not as anticipated, seek medical advice and help immediately.

And, finally, a question of style, lest I be accused of a prejudice I do not harbor: In referring to the victim and rescuer as he (him, and his), I am merely adhering to current grammatical usage, although I have made valiant attempts to use combined pronouns (him/her) where convenient.

Now, with *First Aid for Boaters: The Next Best Thing to a Doctor Aboard,* your first-aid kit, proper gear, good spirits, and a jovial crew, let's set sail with the sincere hope that the only need you will ever have for this book will be to glance at it occasionally, to reinforce that comfortable feeling of knowing help is nearby if the panic button is pushed.

Chapter 1

Crisis, Rescue, and Treatment

Those of you who remember childhood games may recall playing doctor with an imaginary thermometer and stethoscope. In situations of urgency and injury, playing the role of doctor will take on new meaning and a new importance.

First aid is the temporary, immediate care given a victim of an accident or sudden illness on the scene of its occurrence, to lessen his suffering and to sustain him until a doctor can see him. It is very important to know what to do in case you should be faced with such a patient on board ship—and it is equally important to know what *not* to do.

It should be emphasized that substituting for a doctor is never the same as being a doctor, nor will you ever be expected to act with the skill and knowledge of a professional medical doctor when giving first aid. All that can be asked of you, either by the victim or yourself, is that you use the facilities at hand and the available knowledge as best you can.

This book may help you decide and act with greater ease and a little more wisdom; it may help make a difficult situation more comfortable for the victim as well as you by placing some sound advice close at hand, almost as though the doctor were at your elbow. Of course, during your assessment of any crisis there will be times when radio communication with a physician through the Coast Guard or other emergency radio sources may be helpful and necessary. This is emphasized repeatedly throughout the book at especially important and critical moments.

A CRISIS SITUATION

Rescue

It is important for everyone to avoid panic. Give appropriate instructions and take step-by-step actions based on a previously worked-out plan for the management of potential calamities. For example, the man-overboard drill should have thoroughly ingrained into the crew a preplanned series of actions. This is the best protection against panic and the wasted effort of hasty action.

Equipment

Have equipment available for the job at hand. This, of course, includes available line, horseshoe or ring flotation life savers, flotation cushions, overboard flagpoles, flashlights with spare batteries, and first-aid equipment. These are all part of the well-found boat. Know how to use them and always have them ready for use.

The chart below lists the items you will need to stock your first-aid kit. All the medications mentioned here are discussed in the text; many require a doctor's prescription. See chapter 10 for details on how to use them.

MEDICATION	PURPOSE
Analgesics (pain killers)	For pain
Aspirin	For ordinary aches and fever
Nitroglycerin	For chest pains
Talwin®	Emergency treatment for severe pain; by prescription only
Tylenol®	Instead of aspirin
Tylenol® with codeine	For severe pain; wherever aspirin is recommended, Tylenol® may be substituted, tablet for tablet.
Antiallergy drugs and antihistamines	
Actifed®	For nasal decongestion
Adrenalin® (epinephrine)	Emergency drug for severe allergic reaction or intractable asthma; by injection. See page 49 for preparing and giving injections.
Benadryl®	For allergic reaction; as tranquilizer
Chlortrimeton®	Longer-acting antihistamine; less sedating
Antibiotics	For infections. Not necessary on short trips; only when medical help is not available.
Mycolog® ointment	For skin fungus infections
Penicillin	For infections with fever (except bladder infections)
Polysporin® ointment	Skin infections
Tetracycline	Bladder infection; instead of penicillin in case of allergy; when penicillin is ineffective
Antiseptic	For cleaning wounds
Betadine®	Scrubbing antiseptic
Bronchodilators	To dilate bronchi; used for asthma
Bronkometer®	Use only as a last resort
Theolair®	For asthma as necessary
Cough suppressants	For coughs due to colds, postnasal drip
Elixir Terpin Hydrate with codeine	More potent cough suppressant
Robitussin DM®	Eases cough as expectorant

MEDICATION	PURPOSE
Diarrhea control	Antidiarrheal
Pepto-Bismol®	To counteract diarrhea
Lomotil®	To counteract diarrhea
Neotracina®	This medication is not available in the U.S.; over-the-counter in Mexico. Check with doctor on contraindications.
Digestive aids	To counter indigestion
Charcoal, activated	For gaseous distress; also for swallowed poison
Mylanta II® and other antacids	For heartburn, stomach upset, ulcer
Laxatives	To relieve constipation
Dulcolax® suppositories	Laxative
Fleet® enema	To help bowel movement, solution is introduced into rectum
Fleet Phosphosoda®	Laxative; taken orally
Milk of Magnesia	Laxative liquid
Senokot®	Laxative granules
Nasal decongestant	To clear nasal and sinus blockage
Actifed®	Nasal decongestion with antihistamine for head cold and allergy
Afrin® spray	Nasal spray decongestant
Sudafed®	Decongestant without antihistamine
Nausea Control	For seasickness
Antivert®, Bonine®, Bucladin®, Dramamine®	Use as alternatives to Phenergan®
Compazine® suppositories	For intractable vomiting; by prescription only
Phenergan® suppositories and Phenergan D®	For vomiting; by prescription only
Stings	
Poultice (Adolph's meat tenderizer)	For stings of all insects except wasps and poisonous insects
Sodium bicarbonate	For all stings including wasps'
Sunburn and sunscreen lotions	To protect the skin against sunburn or to help relieve burning
Maxifil®, PreSun®	Sunscreen
White vinegar	For sunburn where skin is unbroken

8 FIRST AID FOR BOATERS

MEDICATION	PURPOSE
Tranquilizers Librium® Valium®	For acute anxiety and insomnia
Miscellaneous	
Ace Bandage® Adhesive tape	For sprains and dressings
Airway (Resusitube®)	To keep open airway through mouth to lungs
Band-Aids®	Various sizes for dressing wounds
Betadine®	Scrubbing antiseptic
Gauze (preferably Telfa®), nonadhering	Sterile pads, 3" x 3"—dressings
Inflatable splints	Temporary treatment of bone breaks
Kling® bandage	Self-adhering bandage dressing
Lasix®, 40 mg	Diuretic or water pill
Lip pomade	For chapped lips
Newspaper rolls	Splints for small-bone fractures
Sanitary napkins	For women's menstrual period; can also be used for pressure dressings
Soap—saltwater and freshwater Syringes—2.5 cc. disposable, with ¾" No. 25 needles on each	For injections
Steri-Strips®	To close wound or suture
Thermometer	Measure temperature
Valisone ointment	Steroid (cortisone-like) ointment for itching and irritation of skin

When Victim Is Unconscious

When the victim is unconscious and not breathing, cardio-pulmonary resuscitation may be necessary.

Know your ABCs. (See page 57.)

WHAT TO DO

A. *Airway*

1. Tilt head back while holding neck forward.
2. Remove loose dentures, food, or foreign objects from mouth and throat.

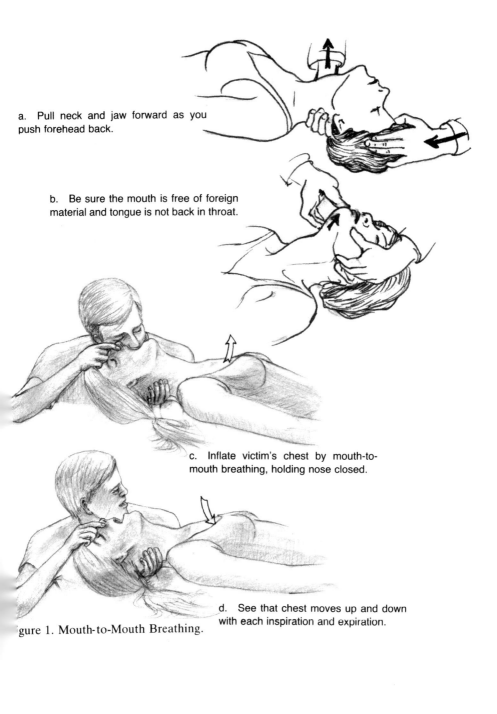

a. Pull neck and jaw forward as you push forehead back.

b. Be sure the mouth is free of foreign material and tongue is not back in throat.

c. Inflate victim's chest by mouth-to-mouth breathing, holding nose closed.

d. See that chest moves up and down with each inspiration and expiration.

Figure 1. Mouth-to-Mouth Breathing.

B. *Breathing*
   1. While holding head tilted back, pinch nose closed (for adult victim).
   2. Place your mouth over entire mouth of victim.
   3. Blow up victim's chest four times in quick succession.
   4. Be sure to see victim's chest rise and start to fall with each of your inflations.
   5. For infants, cover the victim's nose and mouth with your mouth. Remember, it takes less air to inflate a child's chest than an adult's chest.

C. *Circulation*
   1. Feel for pulse over carotid arteries by sliding fingers just to the side of the Adam's Apple and in front of neck muscle.
   2. In child or infant, listen and feel for heart just to left of breastbone.
   3. If no heart action or pulse is found, place victim flat on back on firm surface (not mattress).
   4. Kneel at the side of victim placing the heel of one of your hands on breastbone two finger widths from lower tip of breastbone.
   5. Place the heel of the other hand on back of first hand, keeping all fingers off of the victim's chest.
   6. Now lean forward with your arms straight and vertical and compress the breastbone down toward backbone 1½" to 2" and release.
   7. Repeat this 60 times a minute, once a second, if you are working with a partner who is continuing breathing for the victim.
   8. If you are alone, compress chest 80 times a minute.
   9. If working as a two-person team, the rhythm should be a respiration every 5th chest compression.

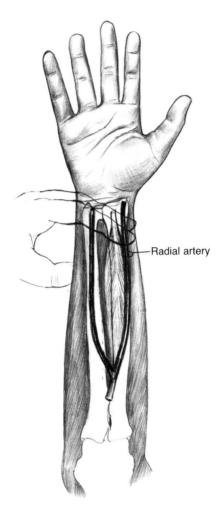

Figure 2. Location of radial pulse at the wrist.

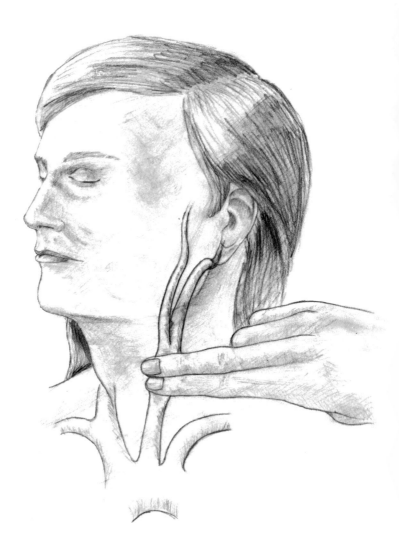

Figure 3. Location of the carotid artery to feel for pulsations with each heartbeat.

CRISIS, RESCUE, AND TREATMENT 13

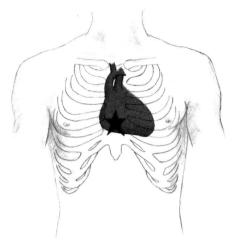

Figure 4. Chest compression. Place heel of one hand one third up from the lower end of the breastbone. Place the other hand on the back of the first hand and press down on the chest with the weight of your body as you shift forward over the victim's chest.

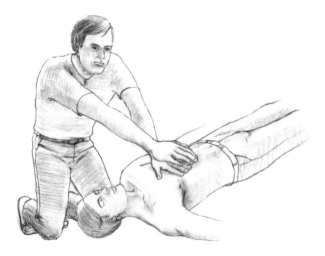

Figure 5. Closed chest compression. Compress the chest using the heel of the hand on the junction of the middle and lower third of the breastbone. *Be sure to keep the fingers off the chest.*

10. Check at carotid artery for pulsation to see that chest compression is effective.
11. If working alone as a rescuer, compress the chest 15 times, then move over and blow up the chest twice rapidly.
12. Be sure to continue the procedure without interruption until help arrives, victim's pulse and breathing are spontaneous, or exhaustion prevents further effort.

Bleeding

The ABCs attended to, make sure that any bleeding is under control. A small amount of blood may seem like a flood to the inexperienced. *Don't panic.* Although spurting blood is usually more serious than oozing and usually indicates arterial bleeding, all bleeding is treated with similar first aid.

What To Do

1. Apply sterile dressing, sanitary pad, or clean cloth over wound.
2. Press down firmly on the dressing until the bleeding stops.
3. Elevate the wound above the level of the heart.
4. Attend to possible shock.
5. For spurting or persistent bleeding see Avulsion (pp. 19–20).

Shock

Shock may take two forms: primary emotional trauma, or fright, combined with injury and exhaustion; and secondary, or physiological, shock.

What To Do

For primary shock:
1. Reassure the victim; sedate or use tranquilizer.
2. Keep the victim warm.
3. Treat the injury.

CRISIS, RESCUE, AND TREATMENT 15

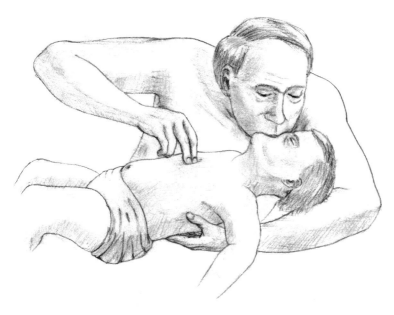

Figure 6. Resuscitation of an infant may just require finger pressure. Remember to place rescuer's mouth over nose and mouth of infant.

These steps will usually be helpful and alleviate the condition.

For secondary shock:
Secondary shock, or physiological shock, is characterized by a drop in blood pressure resulting in cold, clammy skin, mental confusion, and if maintained for a period of time, a noticeable decrease of urinary output. This is a far more serious condition and may be the result of serious blood loss, serious injury to the head, or major injury to the heart or internal organs.

What To Do

1. Elevate lower extremities. This helps blood return to heart.
2. Cover victim. Keep the patient warm.

3. Replace fluids. If the victim is able to drink and keep fluids down, a saline solution consisting of one teaspoonful salt to one full 8-ounce glass of water may be given.
4. Loosen clothing.
5. Adjust position for comfort. Place victim flat out or partially upright if breathing is easier that way.

CHECKLIST:

Having rescued your victim and checked to see that
1. His airway is cleared,
2. His breathing is functioning,
3. His circulation is intact,
4. His bleeding has been controlled,
5. Shock has been considered and attended to,
6. You may now take time to collect your wits.
7. Examine the patient and allow your findings to dictate the next step.

These findings will be discussed in subsequent chapters with action steps to be taken in order, simply stated and described.

Know your limitations and do the best you can.

Chapter 2

The Skin: The First Line of Defense

We rarely stop to realize that the system of our bodies that first confronts the outside world and takes the brunt of attack from all the barbs, sharp edges, bumps, bruises, and stings is our skin. It deserves all the tender loving care we can give it to help it do a better job in protecting us.

Keeping the skin reasonably close to normal temperature and keeping it reasonably dry are, of course, goals to aim for, but they are not always attainable. Forethought is needed before one takes to the sea or woods. Anticipation of weather changes and of the need for changes of clothing is part of good planning. The advantage of being able to store extra clothes in a plastic bag is one of the byproducts of technological advances, and happily so, making it easier to keep something dry and comfortable on board to change into when we finally get off watch and go below deck to warm up.

Assuming that we give it the best of care, what can happen to the skin and what can we do about it?

WOUNDS

A wound is a break in the skin, and ranges from scrapes (abrasions and avulsions) to cuts (incisions), tears (lacerations), and stabs (punctures).

Abrasions

Abrasions are usually referred to as scrapes, or sometimes "strawberries," in which a sliding or scraping injury to the skin may rub off the superficial layers, exposing sensitive underlayers of the skin and perhaps causing some bleeding.

What To Do

1. Scrub thoroughly with a soft cloth or gauze pad and plenty of water and soap or Betadine®.
2. Stop bleeding by hand pressure on sterile gauze, sanitary pad, or clean cloth directly over the wound.
3. Relieve pain with an ice pack on the wound, or aspirin by mouth—two tablets with a full glass of water.
4. If superficial wound, leave open to air.
5. May be dressed with dry Teflon® gauze bandage to protect from rubbing on clothing.

You will note that paints and antiseptic solutions and sprays have not been advised for any of the injuries described. Thorough cleansing with water and Betadine®, an antiseptic cleansing agent, and careful dressing with sterile dressing are considered adequate and appropriate treatment. The addition of other paints, sprays, or lotions is not likely to be of help. In fact, some instances of further injury or allergic reactions to already injured tissue have occurred after the use of such agents. Hydrogen peroxide, if fresh, can be used to irrigate wounds, especially deep or highly contaminated wounds.

Warning. Never wrap an adhesive tape or tight bandage completely around a finger or extremity for fear of cutting off the circulation beyond. If wrapping a pressure dressing (which should preferably be hand pressed), be sure to loosen it at least every ten minutes and apply a loose dressing if the bleeding has stopped. Always look for swelling or blueness of skin and nails beyond the dressing, which would indicate an obstruction to the flow of blood. Loosen the dressing and elevate the extremity.

Avulsion

Avulsion differs from abrasion in that a deeper thickness of the skin is displaced and torn away, exposing subcutaneous or deeper tissues, and usually results in more bleeding. Steps 1, 2, and 3 of What to Do are the same as in Abrasion (page 18). Steps 4 and 5 differ in important ways.

What To Do

1. Scrub thoroughly with a soft cloth or gauze pad and soap or Betadine®, and irrigate with plenty of water.
2. Stop bleeding by hand pressure over sterile gauze or clean cloth on wound (see Warning under Abrasions, above).
3. Relieve pain with an ice pack on the wound or aspirin by mouth—2 tablets with a full glass of water.
4. If an artery is spurting in the wound, pressure should be applied directly over the bleeding blood vessel and held for 10 minutes. Repeat if bleeding continues after 10 minutes of pressure.
5. If this fails, apply pressure with finger or heel of hand over pressure point of artery proximal to injury toward the trunk or heart (see Figs. 7 and 8).
   Warning: Never apply a tourniquet over these points except in the most dire emergencies, such as the case of an amputation or major blood vessel spurting that cannot be stopped by finger or hand

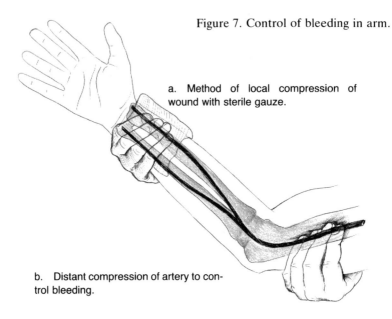

Figure 7. Control of bleeding in arm.

a. Method of local compression of wound with sterile gauze.

b. Distant compression of artery to control bleeding.

pressure. A tourniquet is a band of cloth, rope, or heavy rubber placed around the extremity and tightened by taking turns in the band by rotating a stick placed under the band (see Fig. 9).
6. Elevate wounded part or extremity above the level of the heart.
7. Avulsion may be dressed with dry Teflon® gauze bandage, or antibiotic ointment such as Polysporin® may be applied, then dressed (see Warning, page 19).

Incisions and Lacerations

Incisions are cuts and lacerations are tears in the skin, differing from each other only in the character of the wound. An incision is a sharp knife-like cut in the skin, while a laceration is a jagged tear such as can result from a blow by a blunt object. In either case, the wound may be relatively clean or grossly contaminated.

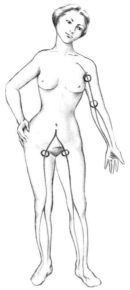

Figure 8. Pressure points for palpating pulses and compressing arteries to assist in control of bleeding.

What To Do

1. Scrub the wound with Betadine® or hydrogen peroxide, and irrigate with plenty of water.
2. Stop bleeding by hand pressure over sterile gauze (see Warning, page 19, against tight wrappings or bandages).
3. Relieve pain with an ice pack on the wound or aspirin by mouth—2 tablets with a full glass of water.
4. If an artery is spurting in the wound, pressure should be applied directly over the bleeding blood vessel and held 10 minutes. Repeat if bleeding continues after 10 minutes of pressure.
5. If this fails, apply pressure with your finger or the heel of your hand over the pressure point of the artery proximal to the injury toward the trunk or heart (see Figs. 7 and 8). Never apply a tourniquet

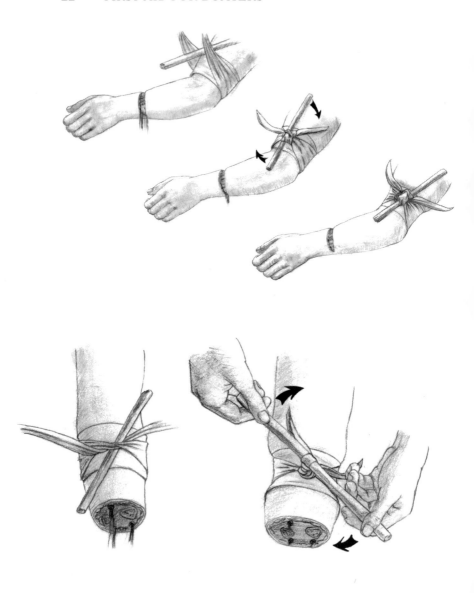

Figure 9. Application of a tourniquet. Apply as indicated for uncontrolled bleeding.

unless you are unable to control the bleeding, as in the case of an amputation or major blood vessel spurting that cannot be stopped by finger or hand pressure. A tourniquet is a band of cloth, rope, or heavy rubber placed around the extremity and tightened by taking turns in the band by rotating a stick placed under the band (see Fig. 9).
6. Elevate wounded part or extremity.
7. Approximate edges of wound and tape in place with Steri-Strips® (narrow sterile adhesive strips) that come in 3- or 4-inch sizes and should be in your first-aid kid.
8. A loose sterile dressing may be placed over wound.

Puncture Wounds

Puncture wounds may result from stabs of sharp objects, from insect bites, sea life, reptile, human, or other animal bites.

What To Do

1. Scrub and irrigate the wound with Betadine® or hydrogen peroxide, and flush with water.
2. Encourage bleeding to irrigate the depth of the wound.
3. Dress with a loose bandage.
4. Obtain tetanus booster with immune human globulin as soon as possible *if not immunized within recent 4 to 5 years.*
   Note: All boaters should have a series of *tetanus toxoid* immunization injections before exposure, *if not previously immunized. A booster is necessary every seven years.* These rarely produce allergic reactions, unlike the old horse serum agents.
5. In case of an animal bite, the animal, if dead, should be examined by a veterinarian, or, if alive, watched for five days under restraint in case of possible rabies. If rabies develops, the health department should be notifed and medical attention sought.

6. For itching of minor bites, apply calomine lotion or a cortisone-type cream or ointment such as Valisone®.
7. Bee stings merit real concern for anyone with a history of sensitivity to stings. There may be a rapid development of allergic reaction symptoms—a rash or hives (large itching welts on the skin), or paleness, faintness, difficulty in breathing, with stridorous sounds (coarse, rough breath sounds), and acute feelings of anxiety and fear.

Bee Sting Allergic Reactions
What To Do
1. Inject adrenalin (a sensitive person should carry ready prepared syringe containing 1 cc of 1–1000 dilution and needle) into the shoulder, arm, or buttock (see chapter 4, page 49, for method of injection).
2. Antihistamine (50 mg Benadryl®) may be given orally or, if feasible, by injection. Repeat every 2–4 hours if necessary.
3. Medical attention should be sought immediately.
4. If sensitivity reaction is not a factor, or as soon as possible, remove the stinger and wash the wound.
5. Apply meat tenderizer in a small moist mound over the puncture site, or make a similar poultice of baking soda.
6. For wasp stings, meat tenderizer will not be effective, so use baking soda.

Venomous Snakebites (Land and Sea) and Poisonous Insects

On shore, poisonous snakes can usually be recognized by a broad arrowhead-shaped head usually wider than the body. An exception is the coral snake, which has a black-tipped head that is not enlarged compared to the rest of the body. It can be recognized by its red, yellow, and black

THE SKIN 25

rings. The bite mark of poisonous snakes will show fang marks outside the row of teeth.

Bites by sea snakes may also be dangerous, and, in fact, poisonous, and should be treated as you would the bite of any venomous snake.

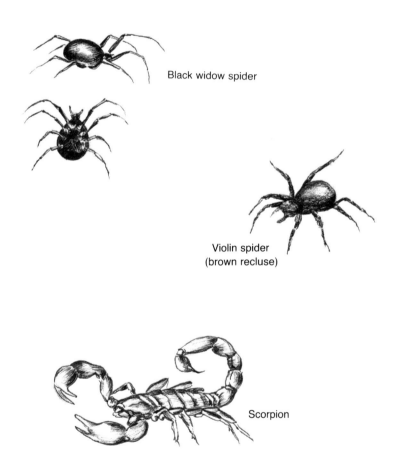

Figure 10. Poisonous insects.

Poisonous insect wounds are most usually inflicted by the black widow spider (a red hour-glass on belly), the brown recluse spider (violin-shaped), or scorpion (with a long, curved tail with stinger on its end). (See Fig. 10.)

What To Do
1. Immobilize the victim and the bitten extremity, with the extremity hanging down if possible.
2. Apply a constricting band (above wound toward the trunk or heart) just tight enough to allow wound to bleed, but do *not* stop pulse beyond constriction. Band may be left on for 30 minutes or until the wound is thoroughly sucked out.
3. Use a blade, sterilized by a flame for a few seconds and cooled.
4. For poisonous snakebite, make an approximately half-inch incision through each fang mark in line with the long axis of extremity and deep enough to go through the skin.
5. Apply suction to the wound either by suction cup or mouth (if there are no open sores) for approximately 30 minutes.
6. Proceed as with puncture wounds (see above).
7. Apply cold pack to wound (ice in cloth or a sack).
8. Seek medical aid. Notify the Coast Guard to obtain antivenom.

Injury by Marine Life

Puncture wounds may be inflicted by marine life such as some species of fish, molluscs, and coral as well as sea snakes. The puncture wounds from the spines, tails, barbs, and other protrusions of sea life may also inject venom into the victim. Unlike insect and snake venom, many of the toxic agents injected by sea life are inactivated by heat.

What To Do
1. Apply constricting bandage as for snakebites.
2. Allow injured limb to hang down.

3. Apply moist packs, as hot as can be safely applied without burning the skin.
4. For pain, give 2 aspirins with a full glass of water or give codeine.
5. Extraction of sea urchin barbs may require medical assistance.
6. Tentacles of a Portuguese man-of-war should be wiped off with a cloth or towel soaked in alcohol.
7. Benadryl® (50 mg) may be given by mouth for sedation or antihistamine effect.

Those swimming or diving in areas of poisonous fish, stinging coral, and sea urchins should learn the appearance and characteristics of these forms of sea life and should protect themselves by wearing gloves, fins, and other protective clothing, depending on the likelihood of contact.

Fishhook Caught in Skin

A fishhook caught in the skin is a frequent emergency situation. It cannot be readily withdrawn because of the barb at the end.

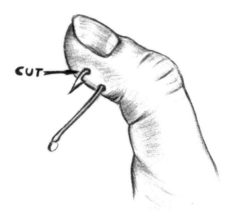

Figure 11. Fishhook embedded in the skin. Sever the barb from the hook with a wire cutter, then withdraw the rest of the hook back through the wound.

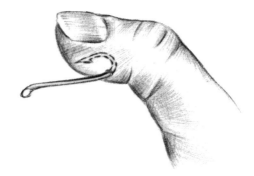

Figure 12. To remove fishhook embedded in the skin, push the barb end through the skin and clip it off with wirecutter. Then withdraw the stem.

What To Do

1. If the barb end is protruding through the skin, sever it with a wire cutter, then withdraw the hook, without the barb, back through the entry tract (see Figs. 11 and 12).
2. If the barb is buried in flesh, grab the stem of the hook with pliers and advance the hook tip through *cleansed* skin with a quick flick.
3. Clean the wound with Betadine® or hydrogen peroxide and irrigate with water.
4. Tetanus booster with human immune globulin should be given as soon as possible.
5. If boil or abscess develops, apply treatment described below.

BOILS AND ABSCESSES

Infections of the skin may result as complications of any of the above injuries. Infection may be recognized by its four cardinal signs: swelling, heat, redness, and pain. In addition, the lymph glands near the wound area draining toward the body or trunk may be swollen and tender, and there may be fever.

Boils or abscesses differ from secondarily infected open wounds in that they may be closed over, representing collections of pus beneath the skin. They may develop from infections of skin cysts or hair follicles, or as complications of puncture wounds.

What To Do
1. Place hot packs (small towel rung out in hot water) over the wound.
   Warning: An exception to this rule is the presence of boils or abscesses around the nose or upper lip. These should be treated with an ice pack and an oral antibiotic (see chapter 10) and referred to a doctor. This is an especially dangerous area for the spread of infection.
2. Wrap saran-type plastic tissue around the towel overlying the infection and tie it in place for 20–30 minutes.
3. Repeat above 3–4 times daily, or more often.
4. If the wound is draining, irrigate it with fresh hydrogen peroxide or a saline solution (one level teaspoon of salt in a full 8-ounce glass of water).
5. If the wound is open and draining, dress with Polysporin® ointment.
6. If the wound is closed over, as in the case of a boil, the hot applications may help bring the infection to the surface, appearing as a gray or white "head." If possible, this should be incised or drained by a physician. Drainage may be accomplished by gentle stabbing with a sterilized needle. The area may be irrigated with a saline solution or hydrogen peroxide as described above and then treated as an open infection.
7. In case of infections with fever and enlarged glands draining from the infected area (they may frequently be felt in the groin or armpit), oral antibiotics (penicillin, 2 tablets 4 times a day) may be necessary and a physician's advice should be sought.

8. The best treatment of fungus infection of the feet (athlete's foot) is prevention by thorough drying of feet, then powder after shower or bath. For skin infections due to a fungus, use Mycolog® ointment or Tinactin® cream or solution twice daily.

Sterilizing instruments: A knife or needle may be sterilized in any open flame—a match, a candle, a lighter, or stove flame. The carbon that collects on the metal can be wiped off with an alcohol sponge. Of course, instruments and water can be sterilized by boiling in a covered container for 20 minutes. Remember to sterilize an instrument, such as forceps or tweezers, with the handle out of the water, or attach a string to the handle so that the sterilized instruments can be picked up without contaminating everything else that has just been sterilized.

BURNS

Burns are a deadly scourge on board ship. In the first place, they can be severe, disabling, and even life-threatening. Secondly, they are almost always a result of carelessness, which is doubly painful to the person responsible.

Burns may result from fires, chemical agents, hot liquids, or electric shocks. They are usually described in degrees according to the depth of the burn area. First-degree burns, or the mildest of burns, are characterized by redness, pain, and mild swelling, as from sunburn or minor scalding. Second-degree burns involve partial thickness of the skin and usually result in blisters. If blisters form, they should usually *not* be ruptured if this can be avoided. Huge coalescing blisters, if uncomfortable, can be pin-pricked with a sterile needle to release the serum. There may be discoloration of the skin and moderate to severe pain.

Third-degree burns penetrate the full thickness of the skin and may appear as blanched white or charred areas. Third-degree burns may be actually less painful than first- or second-degree burns because the nerve endings may be destroyed. At initial examination, it may be difficult, if not

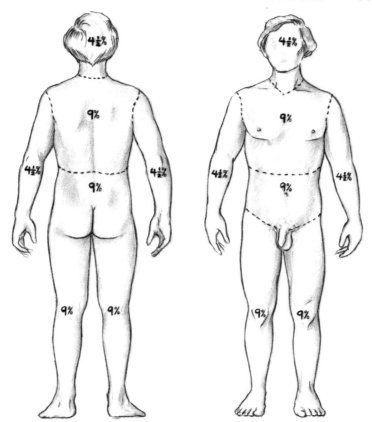

Figure 13. Method of assessing the percentage of the body involved in burns.

impossible, to determine accurately the degree of burn.

Burned areas are also described as percentages of body surface. This can be roughly determined according to the rule of nines, in which an arm is considered 9 percent of the body, the front of the leg and the back of the leg and the head are each 9 percent of the body, and half of the front or back of the trunk is considered 9 percent (see Fig. 13).

In reporting a burn to a physician or the Coast Guard by radio, for example, one should attempt to estimate the degree of the burn and the percentage of body area involved as well as the source or cause of the burn.

What To Do

For first-degree burns:
1. Apply ice or cold packs consisting of clean cloth wrung out in cold water or in white vinegar and water in a ratio of one part of vinegar to three parts of water.
2. Do not place ice directly on burn area.
3. Take pain medication by mouth such as Tylenol® plain or with codeine, as necessary.
4. Antihistamines by mouth such as Benadryl®, 50 mg every 3–4 hours, may be taken for itching and as a sedative.

For second-degree burns:
1. All the above may be used, unless the skin is broken, in which case omit the vinegar solution.
2. If more than 15 percent of an adult body received second-degree burns, seek medical care.
3. With burns about the face, look for injury to eyes or lining of nose, mouth, or breathing tube. If any of these is suspected, the patient should be referred to a doctor as soon as possible.

For third-degree burns:
1. The victim of third-degree burns should receive medical attention and hospitalization.
2. Protect the burned area with a loose, sterile dressing or a clean cloth covering such as a sheet.
3. Cold packs—not ice—may be applied to relieve pain.
4. Elevate the burned limb.
5. Give pain medication as necessary.
6. Encourage fluids by mouth if the patient is conscious and not nauseated. Saline solution, consisting of one level teaspoon of salt in a full 8-ounce of water, is preferable to plain water. Repeat every 30–60 minutes.

7. Observe for breathing distress due to searing effect of inhaled smoke on mucous membranes of nose and throat.
8. Check to see that tongue has not swelled to obstruct airway. Pull jaw forward by bending head back and pushing jaw forward from behind angle of jaw. A plastic airway may be necessary.

Warning: Application of greases, ointments, butter, margarine, or other similar agents is *not* advised. Anesthetic sprays, such as the "caine"-type preparations, can be used, but at the risk of aggravating the condition by a superimposed allergic reaction.

Chemical burns

Chemical burns may result from contact with strong acids or alkalies on the skin or mucous membranes.
1. Irrigate with flowing water or by the "bucketsful."
2. For irrigating the eye, follow step 1 above or, if readily available, use saline solution for irrigation—one level teaspoon of salt per 8-ounce glass of water (see Fig. 14).

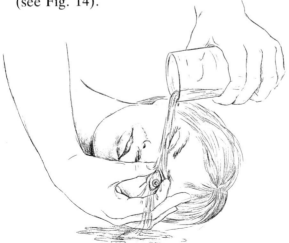

Figure 14. Irrigate the eye to remove foreign object using saline solution.

FROSTBITE

There is both a general systemic and a local, or body, reaction to prolonged exposure to extreme cold. When cold causes local injury or damage to the tissues, as occurs with fingers, toes, and occasionally nose or ears, this is called frostbite. The skin may appear red or blotchy and eventually may turn white as the water in the tissues literally freezes. Gangrene may eventually develop.

What To Do

1. Warm frostbitten areas in lukewarm water (about 100 degrees F.) or cover with blanket or apply mild heat as from the warm body of one snuggled close.
2. Never use extreme heat or a hot-water bottle or bring injured tissues near a fire or hot stove.
3. Do not rub or massage area.
4. Elevate affected limb on pillows or soft support.
5. Move extremity after thawing, but permit no vigorous activity.
6. It is better to wait to defrost area until assurance that reexposure to extreme cold is unlikely, as it is more traumatic to defrost and refreeze than wait to defrost the frostbitten area and maintain warmth subsequently.

Chapter 3

Head Injuries: Beginning at the Top

We shall now plot a course through the human body, pointing out the most likely troubles that might be anticipated.

HEAD

Starting with the head—we mean the one resting on the shoulders—we must first of all be seriously concerned with head injury, especially a blow to the head.

Head Injury: Victim Is Conscious

What To Do

If the patient is conscious,
 1. Question him for signs of confusion by asking about the time and the place where he finds himself. Test for control of the extremities and for balance.

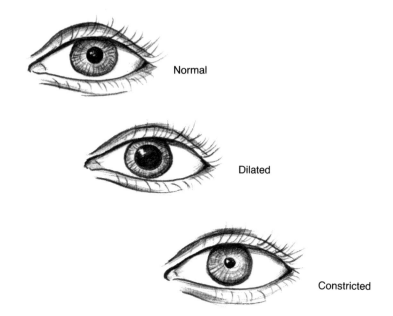

Figure 15. Pupil reactions. Note the size and the reaction of the pupils to light for differences between the eyes and for lack of reaction of the pupil to light.

2. Examine the pupils by lifting both eyelids, looking for any inequality or lack of simultaneous contraction of both pupils after shining flashlight in each eye. (The pupil is the black center of the eye in the middle of the colored ring or iris.) If unequal, or there is a failure to react to light, this is strong evidence of serious injury or stroke and immediate medical attention is necessary (see Fig. 15).
3. Test for weakness of extremities.
4. Aspirin may be taken for headache, but no sedatives or tranquilizers should be given; they can cause symptoms in which injury might be confused with the effects of drugs or a stroke (see step 5).

HEAD INJURIES

5. Continue to observe the victim for drowsiness, increasing headache, or developing coma for at least 24 hours. These symptoms may indicate possible brain hemorrhage or obstruction of brain artery (stroke).

Head Injury: Victim Is Unconscious

Unconsciousness with a head injury is a serious injury until proven otherwise.

What To Do

1. Cover patient and move him or her as little as possible.
2. Consider possible neck and back injury and if suspected, support the spine in a straight alignment.
3. Check skull for defect or laceration. Suspect fracture if there are spreading black and blue areas (bruises) around the eye or behind the ear, or if blood is found in the ears or nose in the absence of a direct blow to these areas. Watery drainage from the nose is also a sign of possible fracture of the base of the skull.
4. If no skull depression or irregularity can be seen or felt, a bleeding scalp wound can be treated by pressure dressing, and cleaned as described in chapter 2, page 21, under Lacerations.
5. Examine the pupils (see step 2, above).
6. When the victim regains consciousness, ask him about his orientation. Does he know who and where he is? Ask him to move all his extremities.
7. If the victim is apparently normal, proceed as directed above under Head Injury: Victim is Conscious. Relapse into unconsciousness is a sign of probable internal bleeding, an extremely serious condition.
8. Repeat step 2 above (re: neck injury) after the patient regains consciousness before allowing him to move, and before releasing support of the neck.

EYES

Foreign Body in the Eye

Dust, a cinder, lint, or an eyelash may find its way into the eye at any time.

What To Do

1. The object may wash out by itself. *Do not rub the eyelid.*
2. To search under the lower eyelid, hold the lower eyelashes and pull the eyelid downward and away from the eye. Ask the patient to rotate his eyes from side to side and upward all the way slowly.
3. To search under the upper eyelid, pull the upper eyelashes out and up after placing a toothpick or wooden matchstick on top of the midportion of upper eyelid. The outer edge of the eyelid may then be folded up and over the stick, after which repeat step 2, except that the eye should be moved down as far as possible instead of up (see Fig. 16, page 39).
4. If a foreign object is found, form a clean paper tissue or soft cloth into a point and just touch it to the object. It should stick to the tissue and be easily removed.
5. If unsuccessful in removing or finding object, prepare a saline solution (one level teaspoon of salt to a full 8-ounce glass of water) and irrigate (pour over) the open eye from the nasal side toward the temple side of the eye with the head tilted, involved eye down (see Fig. 14, page 33).
6. If you are still unable to dislodge the object, place a loose bandage over the closed eye until medical attention can be obtained.

Pinkeye or Conjunctivitis (Infected Conjunctiva)

Pinkeye is an inflammation or redness of the delicate membrane that lines the eyelids and covers all but the front of the eyeball.

HEAD INJURIES 39

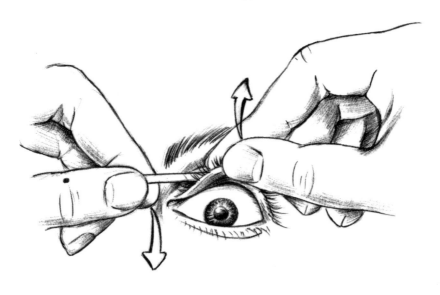

Figure 16. Foreign object in the eye. To search for and remove foreign object from under the upper eyelid, fold the upper eyelid over a match or toothpick.

What To Do

1. Visine® eye drops (or a similar over-the-counter product) may be tried.
2. If there is no response, and in the absence of ophthalmic antibiotic drops or ointment, proceed with eye irrigation (see step 5, above), repeating every 2 to 3 hours.
3. Alternate eye drops with saline irrigation (see step 5, above).

Black Eye or Bruise

The blue-red-purple bruise that appears after, for example, walking into a door is caused by bleeding under the skin. The treatment applies to any bruise or bleeding into the tissues.

What To Do
1. Apply an ice pack (ice wrapped in cloth in a plastic sack) for 20 minutes every hour for approximately 3 hours.
2. Later, hot packs may be applied for 30 minutes 4 times a day.

Snow or Sun Blindness

Snow or sun blindness is caused by insidious overexposure to light usually reflected off snow or water. This is especially common among boaters and skiers and may produce symptoms that may not show up for 12, 24, or 48 hours. Eye discomfort, itching, blurring, a sensation as if a foreign body were lodged in the eye, and pain are the usual symptoms.

The best treatment is time and protection of the eyes from bright light. Bandaging may bring relief. Cortisone-type eye drops may be used. Even better treatment is prevention, by wearing good-quality sunglasses or goggles.

EARS

Earache (Otalgia)

Earache is most commonly due to a blocked Eustachian tube (connects the inner ear and the back of the nose), due to an infection or after descent from a high altitude, or the marked pressure experienced in scuba diving. It may also be due to blockage of the external ear canal (see page 41 below).

What To Do
1. Try yawning, chewing gum, swallowing.
2. If this fails, try holding the nose and blowing against this pressure. While wearing a face mask in skin diving, press the mask against the face and attempt to blow through the nose. Many face masks are equipped with devices for compressing the nose or

obstructing the outflow of air for this purpose.
3. If unsuccessful, use nose spray or nose drops, such as Neo-Synephrine®, ¼–½ percent (see Nose).
4. Follow step 3 with a hot pack over the nose, eyes, and sinuses.
5. Pain medication such as aspirin taken with a full glass of water, or a codeine preparation, may be taken every 4 hours.
6. An oral antihistamine decongestant, such as Actifed®, or a decongestant without antihistamine, such as Sudafed®, may be tried for treatment or for prevention, as in scuba diving (see chapter 10).

Sudden Decrease in Hearing

Sudden deafness may be due to a blockage of the external ear canal where a foreign object or wax is packed in the ear canal. This often follows the use of a cotton-tipped applicator when attempting to clear the ear of wax. Drainage of wax from the ear should be left to the normal process provided by nature. When wax is visible in the external ear, a towel wrapped over the finger can be used to clean it away.

Decreased hearing may also be due to a blocked Eustachian tube (see above).

What To Do
1. With the patient lying on one side, blocked ear up, drop fresh hydrogen peroxide solution into the ear canal until it foams over at the opening.
2. Allow to remain for 5 minutes, then drain by turning head over tissue held over external ear.
3. Repeat 2 or 3 times a day until clear or seek medical help if this treatment is not effective in one or 2 days.

Dizziness

Dizziness may be due to a complication of the blocked external ear or disorder of the internal ear. In case of head injury or in an elderly person it may be a more serious problem and require medical attention.

What To Do
1. Try procedures outlined under either blocked external or internal ear canal (see page 41 above).
2. Give Dramamine®, Compazine®, or Phenergan® suppository every 3–4 hours if nausea or vomiting occurs.

NOSE

Nosebleed

Most nosebleeds usually stop spontaneously and look as if much more blood has been lost than is actually the case.

What To Do
1. If continuous, have the patient sit upright.
2. Place an ice bag over the bridge of the nose with the head tilted back.
3. Place a small roll of gauze (the size of half a cigarette) under the upper lip and press your finger over the lip.
4. If this fails, pack gauze into the bleeding nostril (leave the end sticking out) and squeeze nose. You will, of course, have to breathe through the mouth.
5. If the bleeding stops, leave the pack in place for one to 2 hours before removing carefully.
6. If bleeding does not stop, seek medical attention as soon as possible.

Broken Nose

If the nose appears distorted or crunches on feeling, it is probably broken.

What To Do
1. Apply ice pack over the bridge of the nose.
2. Give pain medicine, usually codeine.

3. Get medical attention as soon as possible.

Stuffy or Blocked Nose

A stuffy nose may be due to a head cold or an allergy. If it is associated with blocked sinuses, it may result in a severe headache.

What To Do

1. Try a decongestant medication with or without antihistamine (see chapter 10).
2. If ineffective, use nose drops such as Neo-Synephrine®, ¼–½ percent, or Afrin®. Tilt the head back over the edge of the bunk so you can see the deck under the head and drop 3–4 drops in each nostril. Stay put for 30 seconds, then slowly pull the head flat on the bunk and remain another minute. If you get up and taste drops, you did not go back far enough or stay down long enough.
3. Nose spray Neo-Synephrine® or Afrin® may be used instead of drops, holding spray nozzle pointing vertically upward and test for spray under light (spray should rise one and one-half to two feet after hard squeeze of bottle). Place each nostril in turn over nozzle so that nozzle points through the top of the head toward the sky, and inhale as you squeeze the bottle.
4. Repeat step 3 in one minute.
5. Nose drops or spray should be used for 2 or 3 consecutive days *only* so as not to injure mucous membranes. After omitting one day, the series of 2 or 3 days may be repeated.
6. After each treatment, a hot pack may be placed over the nose and sinuses to enhance the effect.

MOUTH

Chapped and Sunburned Lips

Chapped lips may be due to dryness of the atmosphere, wind, or sun. Sunburned lips should be treated like a burn.

What To Do
1. Sunburned lips are best treated by prevention, using a sunscreen such as zinc oxide or Maxifil®.
2. Apply lip pomade or Vaseline® for prevention or treatment of dry, cracked lips.
3. Use ice packs for swollen, painful lips.

Dental Problems

Toothache may be due to dental infection or sinus infection.
1. In addition to ice packs and pain medication, a trial with nose spray or drops (see Blocked Nose above) is worthwhile.
2. After suffering a dislodged tooth with a bleeding socket, the socket should be packed with a wad of gauze rolled into walnut size and pressed into the socket by clenching the teeth. Replace the gauze if soaked with blood. When bleeding ceases, do not use the teeth for 12 hours, and encourage drinking carefully (through a straw) so as not to disturb the blood clot.
3. If the tooth is found, immediately clean it thoroughly in a saline solution (one level teaspoon salt in a full 8-ounce glass of water). Squish the saline solution as you would a mouthwash into the socket. Disregard the bleeding.
4. Replace the tooth into the socket, and adhesive tape it in place between the adjacent teeth. An alternative method is to use chewing gum that has been softened by chewing as mortar to fix the tooth in place between the adjacent teeth.

Sore Throat

A sore throat may be symptomatic of anything from shouting too much over the sound of the waves to tonsillitis.

What To Do
1. Gargle every 2 hours with a saline solution (one level teaspoon salt in a full 8-ounce glass of water), being

sure to get to the back of the throat with the
   solution.
2. Soothing lozenges may be tried.
3. If feverish, or enlarged lymph glands are felt in the
   neck below the angle of the jaw, antibiotics may be
   necessary (pencillin, if no allergy to this drug exists).
   Seek medical attention.
4. Aspirin or Tylenol® with a full glass of water should
   be swallowed for pain relief—*not* to be used as a
   gargle. Dosage: 10 grains every 3–4 hours.

Obstructed Breathing

Breathing may be obstructed due to accidental blockage of the throat with bolus of food, or less frequently in adults, swelling of membranes due to inflammation (see Asthma, page 47). Symptoms include choking or coarse noisy, wheezy breathing leading to agitation and panic with clutching of the throat, cyanosis or blue appearance of the skin, and eventual loss of consciousness.

What To Do

1. Try mouth to mouth breathing, carefully covering
   victim's mouth with rescuer's mouth. Note whether
   or not air inflates victim's chest. Be sure to hold
   victim's nose closed when attempting this.
2. If obstruction is suspected, slide finger along inside
   of cheek to back of throat and see if a bolus of food
   can be dislodged.
3. In case of an obstructing bolus of food *that cannot be
   dislodged by finger,* strike the back a firm blow *four
   times.* This is best done by striking *the back between
   the shoulder blades* with the side of the fist.
4. If this fails, a sharp squeeze if the chest, like a "bear
   hug," from behind may dislodge the obstruction.
   This is done by grasping the victim from behind,
   wrapping your arms around the body just *below* the
   ribs. Clasp your fists together in the pit of the
   stomach and give a sharp squeeze of your clenched
   hands in and up under the breastbone (Heimlich

maneuver). This should dislodge the bolus in the blocked breathing tube. The procedure may be repeated if necessary at least three or four times (see Fig. 17).

5. If the victim is unconscious and relaxed enough, the jaw and tongue may be grabbed in a napkin or handkerchief and pulled down to allow one to look at and get to the back of the throat. This may allow one to remove the obstruction with blunt forceps or kitchen prongs.

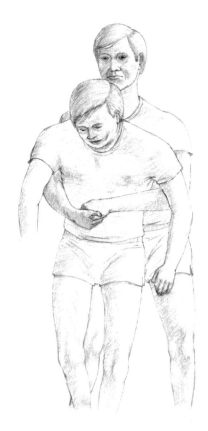

Figure 17. Heimlich maneuver to squeeze out food plugging the windpipe.

Chapter 4

Breathing and Heartbeat: Keep Them Going

Chest conditions may vary from minor and incidental to very critical. In this chapter we discuss some of the more common maladies that might require attention aboard a boat.

ALLERGIES

Asthma

Asthma attacks are frightening for both the victim and observer. They are characterized by a severe shortness of breath with wheezing. The patient usually has more trouble breathing *out* than *in*.

This condition is caused by a spasm of the bronchial tubes complicated by obstruction with dry, thick mucus. It usually occurs in allergic or sensitive people with a family or personal history of allergies. Most frequently, the attack is due to an inhaled allergen, but it may also occasionally follow a bee sting (see page 24), an infection, or emotional stress.

Most allergic patients have had previous experience of these attacks and are knowledgeable about the management of their problem. Many will recognize the occasional onset of an attack associated with stress or an anxiety situation.

What To Do

1. The best prevention and the vital necessity for treatment of asthma is water, taken orally in large quantities. This is a crucial factor and cannot be overemphasized.
2. To further loosen the mucous plugs, an expectorant such as Robitussin® (which is nonprescription) or, better yet, saturated solution of potassium iodide (on prescription) may further encourage the liquefying of the thick mucus.
3. Breathing steam, as from a tea kettle, using a towel for a tentlike collector, may be helpful.
4. A bronchodilator drug such as Theolair®, 250 mg, may be taken every 4–6 hours.
5. Inhaler-type squeeze-bottle treatments such as Bronkometer® may be helpful, but too often the asthmatic patient has been using these inhaler gadgets excessively all along. If tolerance has developed from overuse, they may not be effective at the time of dire need.
6. If all above fails, resort to a suppository of Aminophyllin®, repeated every 3–4 hours if necessary. In a more urgent situation, the injection of Adrenalin® (epinephrine), 0.5 cc, repeated in 15–30 minutes, may be the last resort, indicating an extreme emergency condition requiring medical attention (see below).
7. A dramatic immediate response or relief by any of the above methods of treatment may not be noted. Attempt to keep the patient relaxed, as comfortable

BREATHING AND HEARTBEAT 49

as possible, and sedated with mild tranquilizers such as Valium (5 mg) or Librium (10 mg). With reassurance, these measures will usually be helpful in bringing about a gradual response of the asthma attack.

Injection Procedure
How To Prepare an Injection
1. Break ampule at neck. Protect your fingers by wrapping ampule in gauze square or alcohol sponge.
2. Remove sterile syringe with needle from wrapping.
3. Remove cap from needle and push plunger of syringe all the way in.
4. Insert needle to bottom of ampule.
5. Draw up all the solution into syringe from ampule by pulling back on plunger of syringe.
6. If all the solution cannot be withdrawn because of air in syringe, remove syringe and needle from ampule and turn syringe upside down, needle pointing toward sky. Air will rise to just under needle and can be expelled by gently pushing in plunger of syringe until a drop of fluid appears at tip of needle.
7. To empty ampule, repeat steps 4 and 5 above.
8. Repeat 6 after all the solution has been withdrawn from ampule.
9. Select site for injection in upper outer quadrant of either cheek of buttock (see Fig. 18).
10. Rub area with alcohol sponge.
11. Insert needle using syringe as you would plunge a dart into an orange.
12. After insertion to the hub of needle, hold the syringe in left hand and pull back sharply on plunger with right hand momentarily to see if any blood enters the syringe through the needle.
13. If blood is seen, remove syringe and reinsert at a different spot repeating above procedure.

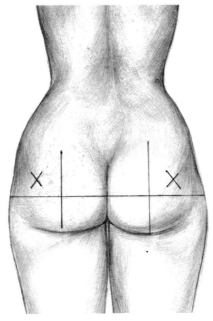

Figure 18. Sites for intramuscular injection. X, the quadrant where intramuscular injections should be given.

14. If no blood is withdrawn into syringe, push plunger slowly until ½ the fluid has been injected through needle.
15. Remove needle by rapid pull of syringe.
16. Wipe area with alcohol.
17. Some medicines such as adrenalin may come as 1 cc solution already in syringe with needle attached. If so, omit steps 1 through 8 and proceed as above with the following exceptions:
    a. Insert the needle approximately halfway in, instead of all the way in.
    b. Inject only one-half the contents of the syringe (0.5 cc), and observe the effect.
18. If symptoms persist or recur in 10–15 minutes, the needle and syringe can be reinserted at another site and the rest of the contents injected.

Anaphylactic Shock

Anaphylactic shock, an overwhelming reaction of the body to an allergen to which it has previously been sensitized, may cause breathing obstruction due to bronchospasm and allergic swelling of mucous membranes (as after a bee sting), with symptoms described under obstructed breathing (page 45). In addition, there is usually severe anxiety with a panicky feeling of impending death.

What To Do

1. Injection of Adrenalin® is needed, which should be in the emergency kit of anyone sensitive to bee stings. This should be injected into the shoulder or arm muscle or buttock, and should be followed by injection of an antihistamine (Benadryl®, 2–5 cc) if available.
2. Seek medical care immediately.

CHEST INJURIES

Fractured Ribs

Fractured ribs may best be diagnosed by noting a painful crunching at the site of most sensitivity on the chest wall following an injury. Occasionally, this can be further confirmed by gently pressing the front and back of the chest, noting consistent pain and/or crunching at the site of injury rather than where the chest is compressed. Breathing may be short because of the pain.

What To Do

1. Pain medication, either two aspirin or Tylenol® or a codeine tablet, every 3–4 hours, should be given as necessary. Always give a full glass of water with aspirin.
2. Rest and inactivity, protecting the chest against further trauma, if possible, is the best method of management.

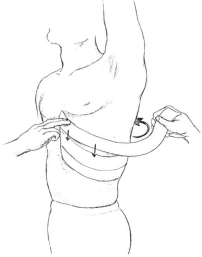

Figure 19. Applying adhesive tape to chest wall restricts painful motion.

3. If physical activity is absolutely necessary, tape the injured side of the chest wall—from midback to midfront and approximately 3 inches below and above the injured area—using an overlapping adhesive tape band 3–4 inches wide (see Fig. 19). Although this may be helpful in permitting moving, it restricts deep breathing and may promote complications in the lungs. Leaving the chest untaped with unrestricted movement is preferable.
4. If the patient coughs up blood or develops a persistent cough or fever, injury or infection in the lung must be suspected and medical attention sought.

Penetrating Chest Wound

An injury puncturing the chest wall through to the space around the lungs is very serious. The victim will be short of breath because the lung on the involved side will collapse. Air may be heard being sucked in and forced out through the wound.

What To Do
1. Cover the wound with a large dressing and attempt to make the dressing as airtight as possible with adhesive tape.
2. Seek medical attention as soon as possible.
3. Give pain medicine and tranquilizers.
4. Reassure the victim and keep at rest.

HYPERVENTILATION

Hyperventilation is perhaps one of the most common breathing disorders and occurs usually in healthy and relatively young individuals. It is characterized by rapid and deep breathing that is clear and free of any sound resembling wheeze or mucus in the breathing tubes. The patient may feel just as uncomfortable sitting, lying, or standing, but is usually very restless and anxious. There may be a sensation of numbness around the mouth and numbness or tingling of the fingers and toes, with gradually increasing stiffness or spasms, eventually ending up as cramps in the extremities and loss of consciousness.

Most frequently, these episodes occur in nervous and anxious individuals and will follow some stress or some anxiety-producing situation.

Aboard ship, one situation occasionally leading to hyperventilation is the well-intended advice given one who is seasick and who is told to take deep breaths. If continued long enough, the whole chain of hyperventilation symptoms may occur. This will differ from a heart attack, pleurisy, injury (other than head injury) and heart failure in that the breathing is clear and deep and is usually free of pain.

What To Do
1. Reassure the patient and give tranquilizers such as Valium® (5–10 mg) or Librium® (10–20 mg).
2. Have the patient lie in a comfortable position, head propped up, and try to keep body temperature reasonably normal by covering as necessary.

3. Loosen all clothing.
4. Keep reassuring and comforting the patient.
5. Have the patient place a paper bag with a cuff rolled down at the top, the size that would hold four or five apples, over the nose and mouth, holding the open end of the bag firmly against the skin so that none of the air in the paper bag escapes around the edges. Have the patient slowly breathe in and out of the paper bag so that the air that fills the paper bag is rebreathed back into the lungs. This will replace the carbon dioxide that has been breathed off by the excessive deep and rapid breathing that causes these symptoms. Paper bag rebreathing may be continued for 5–10 minutes and usually will result in remarkable relief from all symptoms.

CARBON MONOXIDE POISONING

Carbon monoxide poisoning from the fumes of motor exhaust is of serious concern because it can produce confusion, drowsiness, pink skin, and irrational behavior. Irreparable damage or death can result if the victim is not quickly removed from the fumes.

What To Do

Bring the patient to fresh air if carbon monoxide poisoning is suspected.

PLEURISY-PNEUMONIA

An irritation, or injury, or infection of either the outside covering of the lungs or the inside lining of the rib cage (the pleura) will produce a roughened area that will cause sharp, knife-like pain with each breath taken. The symptom is referred to as pleurisy.

There will seldom be any local tenderness at the site of this pain unless the pleurisy is caused by an injury or fracture of a rib. A muscle spasm in the chest wall may also cause an aching or sharp pain with each breath, but not as sharp or severe as true pleurisy.

Pneumonia, or infection of the lung underlying the pleura, may also be a cause of pleurisy or pain with respiration, but is usually associated with cough, fever, and production of sputum that may be green or yellow and occasionally bloody.

What To Do

1. To treat pleurisy, pain medication, usually codeine, should be given every 3–4 hours.
2. Rest and no physical exertion are advisable.
3. Cough medicine may be given, especially cough suppressants mixed with expectorants such as Robitussin DM®, or Elixir Terpin Hydrate with codeine.
4. For fever, two aspirin with a full eight-ounce glass of water every 3–4 hours. If pneumonia is suspected, penicillin in doses of 500 mg, four times a day, may be given if the patient is not allergic and if medical attention is not immediately available to determine more accurately the need for any other selection of antibiotics.
5. The patient should be referred for x-ray of the chest and medical attention as soon as possible.
6. Pleurisy should never be dismissed as inconsequential even if the symptoms subside in a few hours or a day or two, but should be considered a symptom of a potentially serious disease, which requires x-ray and follow-up by a medical doctor.

HEART INJURY

Angina Pectoris

Of all the illnesses that may suddenly befall a member of a boating party, one of the most critical is injury to the heart. This most frequently follows an obstruction of one of the major arteries to the heart (coronary arteries), due either to a blood clot or to the excessive narrowing of a "hardened artery." In the case of a "hardened artery," the blood vessel may be able to carry a sufficient amount of blood for the average needs of the heart, but strenuous activity or severe emotional stress may demand more blood supply than can be adequately provided, and injury to the deprived heart muscle may result.

A mild chest ache in the midchest under the breastbone or in the upper back, usually radiating to the inside of the left arm or perhaps to both arms or the neck or jaw, may indicate a temporary deficiency of blood supply to a portion of the heart muscle. It is usually brought on by exertion, anxiety, or a large meal. This may subside spontaneously and rapidly with rest and relaxation, or by placing a nitroglycerin tablet under the tongue. This condition is called angina pectoris, and usually does not result in damage to the heart muscle.

What To Do

For a patient with a history of angina pectoris with chest pain of a mild degree, the use of nitroglycerin along with rest may be all that is necessary. After subsidence of the episode, the patient is usually able to resume normal activity. He may have repetitions of this type of pain for 20 years or more without serious difficulty.

Heart Attack

If the deficiency of blood circulation is severe enough or lasts long enough to cause heart-muscle damage, the patient is said to have a heart attack. The symptom is usually persistent pain of greater severity, frequently associated with weakness, shortness of breath, perspiration, and much anxiety and fear.

For further explanations of these conditions, with the advice for understanding and prevention, you are urged to contact your local Heart Association office for explanatory pamphlets and literature, or talk to your personal physician.

What To Do

For heart attack, or when heart pain is not relieved by rest and nitroglycerin:
1. Absolute rest in a comfortable position and with reassurance should be the first order. The patient may prefer semisitting to lying flat.
2. If in shock, with perspiration, confusion, and pallor, elevate the lower extremities.
3. Loosen all clothing. Lightly cover the patient.
4. Give pain pills—codeine, 0.5–1 grain, or, if available, Talwin®, 50 mg tablet or injection, every 3–4 hours, or more often if pain is severe.
5. Reassurance and calmness are helpful and to this end tranquilizers such as Valium® 5–10 mg, may be administered by mouth if victim is not nauseated.
6. Oxygen should be breathed if available.
7. Medical attention should be sought as soon as possible.

Cardiac Arrest

The great majority of patients with heart attack will do well with rest, pain relief, and time. Of course, hospital facilities including oxygen and electronic monitoring will improve the outlook immensely.

Occasionally, a heart attack patient may suddenly lose consciousness and cease breathing. The pulse should immediately be checked at the wrist, or carotid area under the angle of the jaw (one side at a time) (Fig. 3), or by listening over the heart with the ear directly on the chest wall (Fig. 20). If no pulse is felt or heart sounds heard, the patient may be considered to have a cardiac arrest or cessation of heart function. Think of your ABCs of closed chest resuscitation. (See page 8.)

What To Do

A. *Airway*
1. Be sure there is a clear airway passage by which air enters and leaves lungs by checking to see that the

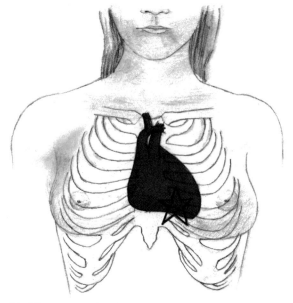

Figure 20. The star marks the area to listen for heart sounds.

      tongue is not folded back into the throat or dentures displaced and obstructing the throat.
2. The head should be tilted back and the jaw pushed forward by pressing forward on the angles of the jaw or back of neck.
3. An airway (plastic, hollow mouthpiece) may be used if available.

B. *Breathing*
1. Breathing must be reestablished and this must be done by mouth-to-mouth resuscitation. Holding the patient's head back and the nose closed, the rescuer literally places his mouth over the patient's mouth and blows up the lungs, using his own breath. Some airways have a tube extending out that can be used by the rescuer to blow directly through the airway into the patient's lungs. Be sure that the victim's

chest is seen to expand as the rescuer blows in to be sure that the effective flow of air is taking place. The mouth-to-mouth breathing should be at a rate of 12 per minute (see Fig. 1).

C. *Circulation*

1. Circulation should be reestablished in the absence of any heart sounds or pulses, by chest compression (see Fig. 4). The victim must be placed on a firm surface, such as a deck or board, rather than in a bunk or bed.
2. The rescuer kneels beside the victim, the heel of his hand placed at the junction of the middle and lower thirds of the breastbone, or two finger widths up from the lower tip of the breastbone. Pressure should be applied, using the weight of his trunk to lean on the breastbone and depress it 1½ to 2 inches. This should be compressed and rapidly released at a rate of 60 per minute or once per second.
3. Mouth-to-mouth breathing takes place every fifth chest compression. This is best done with the rescuers working as a team, but can be performed by a single rescuer alternating between mouth-to-mouth breathing momentarily and the chest compression (see chapter 1, p. 10). The effectiveness of the chest compression, which squeezes the heart, propelling the blood through the circulation, can be checked by feeling for the pulse at the carotid artery just underneath the angle of the jaw. This closed chest resuscitation process should be continued until spontaneous breathing and pulse are noted in the patient or until paramedic rescue squads arrive. The patient may well survive even hours of effective closed chest resuscitation as long as the pupils do not dilate widely and remain fixed when a light is shone in them. Don't hesitate. Don't pause. Keep up your rhythm and you can save a life.

Heart Failure

Heart failure may occur spontaneously or as a complication or result of a heart attack. It represents the backing up of blood behind the heart due to the weakened pumping function of the heart, and produces congestion in the organs, especially the lungs. Increased fluid in the lungs brings on increasing shortness of breath with occasional development of watery, gurgling respiration. The patient will be extremely uncomfortable and agitated, gasping for air and insisting on sitting upright. In some instances, congestive failure may take the form of acute, severe swelling of the lower extremities beginning at the ankles and extending as high as the abdomen. This will be accompanied by severe weakness and sometimes abdominal pain due to swelling of internal organs, such as the liver.

What To Do

1. The patient must have complete rest, propped in a semisitting position with the legs dangling.
2. Medical attention should be immediately sought.
3. Give diuretic or "water" pills to rid the body of excess fluid. The patient may carry these pills himself if he has had a similar problem previously. Some persons may carry diuretic pills in the form of blood-pressure or premenstrual-bloat pills that can be used in such an emergency. One or 2 tablets (such as Lasix®, 40 mg, in the first-aid kit) may be given at a time, repeated every 2–4 hours, depending on their effectiveness.
4. For a patient suffering from shortness of breath, after sitting him or her upright, place tourniquets around the upper part of any three of the four extremities (arms and legs) so that the venous blood return to the heart is obstructed, but the pulses in the wrists and feet are permitted. This may be judged by having the tourniquet tight enough to just barely squeeze a finger under the bandage or wrapping. The tourniquet may be rotated to the unused

extremity releasing one of the tourniquets every 10 minutes in a continuous rotation. Tranquilizers, and, if available, Talwin® or codeine, every 3–4 hours as necessary, may be given.
5. Even if the shortness of breath subsides, the symptoms should be considered urgent, and the possibility of a silent heart attack or irregular heart rhythm searched for by a medical doctor as soon as feasible.

DROWNING

For a victim who has inhaled water, the problems divide themselves into immediate and delayed (see also chapter 9, page 102).

What To Do

1. If victim is not breathing, proceed with ABCs of closed-chest resuscitation (see page 57).
2. Watch for vomiting, and be sure to turn unconscious victim on his side and allow vomitus to drain out rather than into lungs.
3. Treat for shock (see page 13).

Six to 12 hours after the episode a new danger may develop from absorbed water from the lungs getting into the circulation.

What To Do

1. If near-drowning was in salt water, give diuretic (water pill) such as Lasix®, 40 mg, every 2–4 hours for 3 doses until medical advice is available.
2. Encourage intake of orange juice if patient can tolerate oral fluids.
3. If near drowning was in fresh water, do not give diuretic, as the purpose of this medication is to remove excess salt in the system, which is not a problem in fresh water.
4. If the patient is not allergic, and further medical care is delayed, start penicillin, 2 tablets every 6 hours.

Chapter 5

The Gastrointestinal Tract: Above and Below the Belt

The gastrointestinal tract consists of the hollow tube that starts at the mouth and ends with the anus; it includes all of the esophagus, stomach, and intestines that lie in between. This system also includes the liver, gallbladder, and the various organs that produce digestive juices (the pancreas, salivary glands, etc.). (See Fig. 21.)

Disorders of the mouth and swallowing were discussed in chapter 3, pages 43–45.

POISONING

Poisoning by Toxic Material

Before getting into specific areas of the gastrointestinal tract, let us discuss poisoning, which most frequently results from swallowing toxic material, often household materials such as paints, turpentines, detergents, acids, or alkali solutions. Drugs swallowed in excess can of course produce a variety of serious and perhaps fatal effects. Food poisoning may result in toxic effects, due either to food going bad (most likely from bacterial contamination), or by the toxicity of the food itself (for example, certain kinds of fish). Some of the agents that are toxic when swallowed, such as industrial chemicals, may also be dangerous because of inhaled effects, producing lung complications or allergic reactions.

What To Do

1. In general, in cases of any kind of poisoning, remnants or evidence of the nature of the poison should be retained.
2. If the patient vomits, some of the vomitus should be collected for analysis and the patient referred for medical care.
3. In any case of serious poisoning, a call should be placed to the nearest poison center, which can be reached through the Coast Guard or city or county health agencies or hospitals. There advice regarding management may be obtained.

For immediate first aid, however, there are a number of steps that can be taken at once.

1. Encourage the victim to swallow large quantities of liquids; an adult should drink three or four glasses of water or milk.
2. Encourage vomiting by tickling the back of the throat with some object such as a spoon or handle of a toothbrush.
   Warning: If a corrosive agent such as strong acid, alkali, gasoline, or turpentine has been swallowed, do not induce vomiting, but instead give large quantities of water with four ounces of mineral oil or the white of an egg. If acid has been swallowed, one should give an antacid such as 2 or 3 ounces of Mylanta II® to try to neutralize the acid, or if a

strong alkali solution is taken, such as lye, a dilute vinegar, orange, or lemon juice solution should be used in an effort to neutralize the alkali.
3. Keep the airway open, using a plastic airway if necessary, if the victim is unconscious or paralyzed.
4. Keep the patient turned to the side and lower the head below the level of the chest if the patient does vomit to prevent inhaling of the vomitus.
5. Treat for shock by keeping the patient at rest, warm, legs elevated, and reassured as much as possible.
6. Look on the label for recommended antidote. If there is none, try activated medicinal charcoal. Approximately 3 ounces should be taken with milk or water in an effort to absorb the poison.
7. If excessive amounts of tranquilizers or sedatives were ingested, black coffee may be taken if the patient is able to swallow.
Warning: Do not give anything by mouth to a victim who is unconscious.

Poisoning by Contaminated Food

Contaminated food usually means food in which bacteria have grown. This usually results in severe cramps with diarrhea and/or vomiting.

What To Do

1. If diarrhea is the major symptom, give the patient Lomotil®, one or 2 tablets every 4 hours.
2. Kaopectate® or Pepto-Bismol®, two tablespoonsful every ½ hour for 4–6 doses, will absorb some toxins and water.
3. Encourage the patient to drink fluids, especially orange juice or tomato juice if they can be tolerated (if the patient is not nauseated or vomiting). If there are symptoms of severe dehydration (severe thirst, dryness of the tongue, throat, and skin) from previous inability to keep down fluids, give saline solution consisting of one level teaspoonful of salt in

an 8-ounce glass of iced water, to be sipped as rapidly as possible at one- to 2-hour intervals. (Instead of the saline solution, a level teaspoonful of salt may be added to an 8-ounce glass of tomato juice.)
4. If vomiting is a major factor, rectal suppositories such as Compazine® or Phenergan® may have to be given every 2 to 4 hours until oral medications and fluids can be taken.
5. When symptoms are persistent or do not respond to the above measures, serious dehydration and potential shock require that medical attention be sought.

Poisoning by Ingestion of Toxic Fish

Some fish or shellfish can cause serious toxic effects by bacterial contamination, from intrinsic poisons, or from allergic reactions.

What To Do
1. Seek medical attention, preferably in the area where the incident occurs, since there is apt to be more information about the local toxic or poisonous fish or the status of the shellfish in that area.
2. The symptoms may be treated as outlined in the section on contaminated food (page 64).
3. Prevention is the best measure. Check in advance with local sources for information on the safety of eating certain kinds of fish or shellfish in that area and during that season.

DIGESTIVE DISORDERS
Indigestion

An excess of acid and gas in the stomach, sometimes aggravated by spasms of the emptying end of the stomach (the pylorus), usually causes indigestion. There may be a tendency for the acid stomach contents to be partially regurgitated up the swallowing tube or esophagus, producing what is referred to as heartburn or waterbrash. This may be aggravated by highly seasoned foods, coffee, alcohol, or by some specific food sensitivity of the individual.

What To Do
1. Treat with antacids such as Mylanta II® in the dosage recommended on the label—taken, however, at one-half to one hour intervals, or less frequently, depending on the symptoms.
2. Antacids may be taken prophylactically, approximately one hour after a meal, if there is a tendency for recurrent stomach distress. In this case, referral to a medical doctor for further diagnosis and treatment is advised. This condition may best be treated by prevention, which should include eating one's meal in as relaxed a manner and as slowly as possible, sitting up rather than lying down immediately after the meal, refraining from strenuous physical activity, if possible, immediately after eating, and restricting the intake of irritating or allergenic foods.
3. If these symptoms tend to awaken the patient at night, peptic ulcer or esophagitis (inflammation of the esophagus) should be considered. A trial of Mylanta II® at bedtime, along with elevation of the head of the bed or bunk, so that the person will tend to sleep at a slight slant from head down to the legs, may be helpful. Adequate medical examination should be done as soon as possible.

Peptic Ulcers

Peptic ulcers most commonly occur in the duodenum—the tube that empties the stomach. Ulcers also may occur in the stomach itself; in this case the possibility of cancer must be considered and should be ruled out only by medical examination and persistence of treatment to the point of complete healing. Duodenal ulcers tend to recur and occasionally bleed varying amounts of blood, from a minimal to a life-threatening hemorrhage.

What To Do
1. If vomiting with blood occurs, or if bowel movements contain black, tarlike stools, immediate medical attention should be sought.
2. For ulcer pain, which is usually a burning sensation located in the upper-middle or right-middle upper abdomen, take antacids such as Mylanta II® every 2 hours, or more frequently, if necessary, drinking a glass of milk on the alternating hour. This should be effective and should be continued around the clock.
3. Meals may be incidental to the above for the victim of acute ulcer pain and should consist of soft, bland food such as hot cereal, soft hamburger, soft-boiled eggs, cottage cheese, etc. Alcohol, coffee, spicy foods, and smoking should be avoided.
4. Four or five small meals a day are preferable to one or two larger meals. Anyone with ulcers or a history of ulcers should always examine bowel movements (stools) for a black, tarry appearance as the first indication of possible bleeding unless, of course, medications or foods high in iron (such as raisins or spinach in large amounts) have been eaten.
5. Rupture of an ulcer is a dreaded complication, with widespread abdominal pain (occasionally felt also in the shoulder tips), boardlike, rigid stomach wall muscles, and the appearance of a severely ill person. See Acute Abdominal Pain, pages 69–75 below. A physician should be sought immediately.

Gastroenteritis

This is commonly referred to as the "GIs," and represents a condition similar to food poisoning. However, it may be due to a virus or even an emotional upset.

What To Do

See the section on food poisoning (page 64) for symptoms and management.

Constipation

The best treatment for constipation is prevention, which can almost always be simply done by assuring an adequate intake of fluids. In hot or humid weather, six to eight glasses of liquids other than coffee should be consumed daily, and in cooler weather, four to six glasses of fluid which, of course, may include all liquids drunk other than coffee or caffeine-containing fluids. The latter tend to act like diuretic pills in promoting increased urination and passing off increased amounts of fluids through the kidneys.

In addition to fluids, it is necessary to have adequate roughage in the diet, which can be provided by eating an orange or two a day, excluding pits and skin, but including the pulp. Half a grapefruit, twice a day, is an acceptable substitute. Bran flakes and similar bran cereals may also be used to improve bulk ingestion. In the absence of any of these available sources of bulk, preparations such as Metamucil® or Konsyl® should be taken as directed on the container.

What To Do

Once constipation has developed, there are several steps that can be taken:
1. Milk of Magnesia, 2–4 tablespoonsful, may be taken as necessary.
2. If bowel movements are hard and hemorrhoids tend to be a problem, an occasional dose of mineral oil, one to 2 tablespoonsful, may be used, but mineral oil should *not* be taken on a daily basis because it tends to wash out important vitamins and nutrients.
3. If preferred, a preparation such as Senokot® taken as tablets or granules may be found more acceptable or effective.
4. If all the above measures fail, then Fleet's Phos-

phosoda® may be taken (by mouth) or a Fleet® enema (rectally) as directed. The enema may be most advantageous on board a boat because it takes effect within a few minutes, rather than risking the possibility of frequent bowel movements at some less convenient time.

Diarrhea

Food poisoning or infection or simply an overdose of laxatives may result in diarrhea. In any case, the major danger is dehydration and, of course, the inconvenience is a problem.

What To Do

1. Lomotil®, one or 2 tablets every 3–4 hours, will usually be effective in slowing down or stopping the bowel movements.
2. Kaopectate® or Pepto-Bismol®, 2 tablespoonsful every 2–3 hours for 4–6 doses, is helpful.
3. Hydration must be maintained by increased fluid intake, preferably orange juice or tomato juice to replace some of the elements lost in the diarrhea.
4. Boiled rice, bananas, and tea are a good diet while this disorder lasts.
5. If blood is noted in small quantities, especially in streaks, with hard bowel movements, it may not be immediately ominous, but should be brought to the attention of a physician at the earliest convenient time. The occurrence or persistence of gross bleeding, however, may indicate a medical emergency and a physician's attention should be sought as soon as possible.

ACUTE ABDOMINAL PAIN

Almost any organ in the abdominal cavity can be implicated as the cause of acute abdominal pain. We will discuss them in, roughly, their decreasing order of frequency.

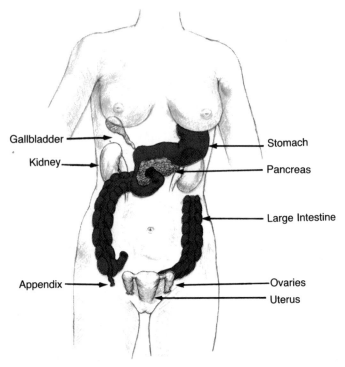

Figure 21. Location of abdominal organs that are common sources of pain.

Mittelschmerz

A ruptured ovarian follicle is one of the most frequent causes of acute abdominal pain in females. Every month, unless the woman is taking contraceptive pills, an ovum or egg ruptures out of the ovary on one or the other side. This is occasionally accompanied by slight bleeding and may produce varying amounts of pain in the lower abdomen on the side of the ruptured follicle. If pain is on the right side, it may be confused with appendicitis. Vomiting seldom accompanies this disorder. The onset is usually abrupt, occurs approximately midway between periods, and the patient may recall having numerous similar episodes in the past, making appendicitis much less likely.

What To Do
1. If in doubt, seek medical advice and examination.
2. Treat with pain medications as necessary.
3. Ice pack over painful area of abdomen.

Appendicitis

Appendicitis may start as a dull pain anywhere in the abdomen, especially in the upper or mid abdominal area, and is usually constant. Over the hours, it may work its way gradually to the right lower quadrant of the abdomen and become more severe and tender to pressure. Vomiting may occur, but seldom more than once. The temperature may be elevated to approximately 100 degrees F. orally or may be subnormal.

What To Do
1. This course of symptoms is strongly suggestive of appendicitis and should be referred for medical attention as soon as possible.
2. If appendicitis is even remotely suspected, do *not* give laxatives.
3. Pain medicine may be given if medical attention is not immediately available.
4. An ice bag may be placed over the area of greatest pain and tenderness.

Acute Gallbladder Disease

Gallbladder disease may be due to inflammation, infection, or passage of a stone that may be obstructing. This pain is felt slightly higher in the abdomen on the right side and may go through or around to the back opposite the anterior right upper quadrant of the abdomen. This pain can be rather steady and constant but may wax and wane irregularly. There may be more frequent vomiting and higher fever. There is usually a history of indigestion or difficulty in eating foods in the cabbage family such as cauliflower, brussels sprouts, and broccoli, as well as raw apples and fatty foods. A previous history of known gallstones could be further suggestive information.

What To Do
1. Gallbladder disease requires medical attention.
2. Codeine or Talwin®, every 3–4 hours, may be given temporarily until medical attention is available.
3. Ice packs may be helpful over the painful area.

Acute Pancreatitis

Acute pancreatitis may be a very serious disease characterized by severe pain in the upper abdomen with boardlike, rigid abdominal muscles and great tenderness to percussion or tapping the back opposite the area of pain in the upper abdomen. The patient may writhe or roll from side to side, unable to lie still with the pain. He may well have had a number of alcoholic drinks and a heavy meal just before the onset of the attack. The patient may vomit repeatedly and have a high fever and will be very sick.

What To Do
1. Patient will require immediate and urgent medical attention.
2. Pain medication should be given preferably by injection.

Kidney Stone

The pain of passing a kidney stone may be the most severe of any, usually starting in the back on one side or the other, and radiating around the flank toward the groin. If urine is passed, it may be smoky in appearance or grossly bloody. The pain may come intermittently, as the stone passes down the tube from the kidney to the bladder. It will let up rather suddenly with remarkable relief as the stone finally enters the bladder. Sometimes if the stone remains stationary for a period at one place in the tube emptying the kidney (ureter), the pain may subside until the stone starts to move again.

What To Do
1. Although the pain is severe, passing a kidney stone is seldom an emergency if the pain can be relieved

by medication (codeine or Talwin®).
2. Passage of the stone may be encouraged by taking oral fluids.
3. If fever develops, the situation now becomes complicated and should be referred for medical attention as soon as possible. Tetracycline should be started if fever is present.

Acute Muscle Strain

A muscle strain of the abdomen may mimic any of the disorders of the internal organs. On palpating or pressing the abdomen, however, one may be surprised to see how deep one may press without producing any significant tenderness.

The symptoms may be reproduced by having the patient lift his or her head or legs or both at the same time off the bunk or bed while feeling the tensed abdominal muscles. When the symptoms can be reproduced by this simple maneuver, this is most likely a case of a simple muscle strain rather than any serious internal disorder.

What To Do

1. Treat with hot packs to abdomen.
2. Take pain pills.

Gas Pocket

Gas blocked behind a section of bowel in spasm may produce recurrent abdominal cramps. This is one of the most severe pains of all and is due to the distended loop of bowel. It might result from an intestinal obstruction, but more often it is due to a temporarily blocked bowel, as in spasm or in constipation.

What To Do

Where there is distention of the abdomen and a history of constipation or bowel spasms or cramps, most gratifying relief can be achieved by providing a Fleet® enema, promoting a bowel movement and immediate relief. A Fleet® enema is a medication contained in a disposable plastic bottle with a nozzle that is inserted into the anus, introducing the fluid into the rectum. The patient should preferably be lying on his left side. The effects can be noted within 5 or 10 minutes.

This may save the day for many a cruise or trip that would otherwise be broken up by concern that there is a medical emergency. Certainly a Fleet® enema should be in any first-aid kit where more than one day of travel is expected.

Ruptured Peptic Ulcer

Ruptured ulcer is described on page 67.

What To Do

1. Immediate medical attention is needed.
2. If a ruptured ulcer is suspected, give nothing by mouth.
3. Place ice pack on abdomen.
4. If available, Talwin®, 50 mg, may be given by injection.

Seasickness and Hangovers, see chapter 8.

CHECKLIST:

To manage a patient with acute abdominal pains:
1. Examine the patient, looking for the indicators and signs described above before giving any significant amount of pain-relieving drugs so as not to confuse the picture.
2. If patient is not nauseated or vomiting, codeine, 0.5–1 grains, or Talwin® tablet every 3–4 hours may be given as necessary for pain.
3. An ice pack may be placed over the most sensitive or painful area and should be left on 30 minutes at a time, and placed again every 15–30 minutes if the pain does not subside.
4. In most cases, unless diarrhea or severe dehydration are factors, a minimum amount of fluid should be given by mouth. Sucking on a moistened cloth or

occasionally on ice chips may be helpful for the patient who feels parched and thirsty and should not take anything by mouth.
5. In case of dehydration from previous diarrhea or vomiting, see the section on the management of food poisoning, page 64.
6. In most cases of severe abdominal pain, medical advice will be necessary.

Chapter 6

The Genitourinary System: When the Plumbing Goes Bad

There are a few disturbing and sometimes frequent or critical problems that can develop, even on a short cruise, in the reproductive and urinary organs. Knowing how to interpret their seriousness and what initial steps to take in their management may make the difference between an interrupted trip and a short period of discomfort.

PROBLEMS OF THE URINARY SYSTEM

Urinary Retention

The inability to empty a full bladder is a distressing occurrence especially frequent among older men with prostate disease. This may also occur, however, in anyone with infection of the lower urinary tract and, sometimes, from embarrassment due to lack of privacy. Some helpful steps that can be taken:

What To Do
1. Recognize the possibility of embarrassment and attempt to provide privacy as much as possible.
2. Allow water to run in spigot as a starter, or pour sea water from bucket into sink or head.
3. If this fails, pouring water over genital organs is often effective.
4. Sit in a hot shower or tub and relax—even urinate right in the water. One can always wash off afterward.
5. If none of the above measures are helpful, seek medical help for catheterization or draining bladder through needle puncture through the lower abdomen.

Bladder Infection

Perhaps one of the most common disorders that occur in women is bladder infection. This is characterized by a frequent and urgent sense of a need to urinate, burning as urine is passed, and, occasionally, fever. It may be a recurrent disorder or a first-time occurrence. It usually represents an infection of the bladder or the urethra (the emptying tube of the bladder).

What To Do
1. Encourage intake of large quantities of fluids—up to eight glasses a day.
2. If patient is not allergic to the drugs, tetracycline, 2 capsules 4 times a day, or 2 penicillin tablets, 3 to 4 times a day, will usually be helpful.
3. If patient is allergic to both or is not responsive, medical attention should be sought.
4. If urethral or vaginal discharge is noted, venereal disease may have to be considered. Even if the discharge clears up after a course of antibiotics, a follow-up visit to a doctor is urgently advised.

Kidney Stones

See page 72.

PROBLEMS OF THE REPRODUCTIVE SYSTEM

Excessive Vaginal Bleeding

The most common cause of excessive vaginal bleeding is a heavy menstrual period, which is usually self-limiting. It may occur with changes in activity or environment. In pregnancy, bleeding may represent a spontaneous miscarriage, and if products of conception are seen, this, of course, becomes obvious.

What To Do

1. Have patient lie flat in bunk or bed to rest as quietly as possible.
2. Apply ice pack to the lower abdominal area.
3. If bleeding persists, seek medical care.

Injury or Infection of the Contents of the Scrotum

Both the testes and the associated duct system, called the epididymis, are subject to injury or inflammation. In either case there may be painful swelling.

What To Do

1. Rest is necessary to prevent further trauma and discomfort.
2. The scrotum should be elevated on an ice pack (ice in a plastic sack wrapped in a cloth) placed between the legs, or else the scrotum may rest on the back of a strip of adhesive tape, 3 or 4 inches wide, stretched across both thighs just under the scrotum. An ice bag may then rest against the scrotum—*not on top!*

Chapter 7

Musculoskeletal Injuries: Those Dry Bones

Musculoskeletal injuries include bone fractures and dislocations as well as strains and tears of muscles, ligaments, joints, and tendons. Most of these are due to trauma, and too often that means carelessness.

Since the best treatment is prevention, an attitude of caution and anticipation of possible danger is part of good seamanship. Planning for good footing, placing nonskid material on stairs, clearing lines and equipment from underfoot, and keeping a neat and trim ship will go a long way toward prevention.

MUSCLE INJURY

Persistent spasm and swelling in muscles are most likely due to bleeding or fluid in the muscle, and are usually associated with tearing or stretching of muscle fibers. This may occur after surprisingly small amounts of stress in a muscle that is poorly conditioned or ill-prepared for strain. Crush injury to muscles usually results in more severe damage.

What To Do
1. Elevate the arm or leg if this is the area of injury.
2. Apply ice packs. Place ice in a plastic bag, and wrap both in a towel or cloth.
3. Wrap the injured muscle with an elastic bandage, not too tightly because its natural inclination to swell against a tight dressing may constrict blood vessels, injure nerves, and impair blood supply or nerve function beyond the wrapping.
4. After the first 12 to 24 hours, hot packs may help increase the rate of absorption of the blood clot (hematoma) or fluid.
5. When considering the possibility of fracture, look for bony tenderness, a crunching sound or deformity during examination.

JOINT SPRAINS

Sprains are usually acute injuries around joints resulting from stretching or tearing of ligaments. The major concern is that a fracture may have occurred, which may require an x-ray to be sure whether or not this is the situation. If fracture is ruled out or felt to be unlikely:

What To Do
1. Elevate the arm or leg if that is where the sprain occurred.
2. Apply an ice pack.
3. Take pain tablets.

4. When reasonably relieved of acute pain, begin gradually to use the arm or leg as normally as possible.
5. If the area is too painful to use, rest, and elevate the involved extremity with ice packs on for 30 minutes, and off one to 2 hours for the first 24 hours.
6. If fracture is unlikely and the injured limb must be used, wrap the injured joint with Ace®-type elastic bandage. Start beyond the injury and wrap toward the trunk.
7. Check for blue skin color, swelling, and obstructed circulation beyond bandage, and loosen if necessary.

DISLOCATIONS

Dislocations are ends of bones that come out of joint. This occurs most commonly in finger, toe, and shoulder joints.

What To Do

A steady, firm pull on the extremity or appendage will frequently help replace the bone in the joint. If you are unsuccessful at the first pull, it would be better to leave well enough alone, and splint the dislocated joint as described below in Fractures.

FRACTURES

General Measures for the Care of a Patient with a Fracture

A positive diagnosis of a fracture may be made when there is evidence of gross deformity and, occasionally, on palpating a tender or painful area, where a crunching may be felt as fragments of bone rub against each other. There is usually immediate swelling and discoloration at the site of a fracture.

It is neither reliable, as a test, nor advisable to permit the patient to see whether he can carry his weight or manipulate the involved part, even fingers or toes, since a fracture can occasionally allow for a surprising amount of mobility and function, and hence give false reassurance. When in doubt, treat the injury as a fracture until medical attention and x-rays are available.

Fractures are generally subdivided into closed and open fractures, depending on whether the skin is broken at the site of the wound.

What To Do

1. Relieve pain with codeine or Talwin® tablets as necessary.
2. Attempt to allow for as comfortable a position as possible while maintaining rigid splinting and immobility of the fracture site.
3. Sedate as necessary with tranquilizers such as Valium, 5–10 mg, every 3–4 hours.
4. Ice packs may be applied over fracture site if fracture is closed—that is, the skin is not broken—and over a sterile antibiotic ointment dressing where an open fracture has occurred.
5. General care should also include management of primary or neurogenic shock. This is due to anxiety and emotional reaction as well as the physical trauma the body receives at the moment of an injury sufficiently severe to produce a fracture. Shock should be treated by keeping the patient warm, elevating extremities, and by reassurance.
6. Splinting. This may tax the ingenuity of the rescuer, and requires some anticipatory planning for shipboard. Inflatable splints are available that pack flat when deflated and fit into a small space. The adult-sized splint is the most practical. In other situations, rolled-up newspapers, slats of wood, or appropriate-sized lengths of board may be used. On occasion, a small pillow or towel may be rolled up or folded so as to serve as an adequate splint, especially for small bones. Techniques will be described later.

MUSCULOSKELETAL INJURIES 83

Closed (Simple) Fractures

A. The Extremities

What To Do

1. After determining the probable fracture site, attempt to splint the joint above and below the site of fracture.
2. Pad all bony prominences before binding splinting material, such as wood or even a hard newspaper roll. Felt or other soft material wadded up may be used. Be especially careful at elbow and knee.
3. In the absence of any other source of splinting material, a broken leg may be splinted to the uninjured leg, again being sure to pad between prominences such as the knees and ankles. The splinting material such as newspaper or inflatable bag or board may be held in proper alignment by tying strips of bandage or torn strips of sheet at close intervals the entire length of the splinted area. (This process may be performed over the clothing, which will add further padding and protection against the rubbing or trauma effect of the splint.) (See Fig. 22.)

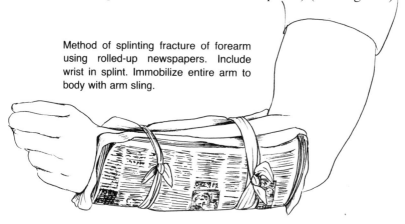

Method of splinting fracture of forearm using rolled-up newspapers. Include wrist in splint. Immobilize entire arm to body with arm sling.

Figure 22. Splinting for forearm.

4. While adjusting a splint and tying it in place, one person should keep a steady gentle pull on the extremity in the direction of separating the fracture ends, if skin over fracture is unbroken (see Open Fracture). For open fractures care must be taken not to withdraw the bone fragments deep into the wound by traction (see page 82).
5. For fractures of the upper and lower arm as well as the elbow and shoulder joint injuries, the arm may be supported in a sling arrangement and then further fastened to the chest wall by wrapping the entire extremity and sling to the chest in order to maintain immobility (see Fig. 23).
6. Hands and fingers are best splinted over a ball, or a rag wadded up into a ball, to maintain the fingers in a curved, rather than a straight, position.
7. After adjusting splints, some swelling of the extremity may be noted and, occasionally, blue-purplish coloring. Be sure to *check at repeated intervals* for signs of coldness or pallor or lack of pulse in the area beyond the fracture or splint site; also check by pinching the toe or fingernail to see whether it produces blanching (whiteness) that doesn't return to pink when released. These findings indicate an obstruction of the blood flow due to bandaging that is too tight or compression of the splint against a major blood vessel. If these symptoms are seen, loosen the wrapping enough to allow blood to circulate and color, warmth, and pulse to return.
8. Elevate the injured extremity above the level of the heart to reduce pain and swelling.

B. Collarbone

What To Do

A broken collarbone is treated best with a figure-eight strapping. This is done by wrapping an elastic bandage across the shoulder toward the front, then under the armpit, and across back to the opposite

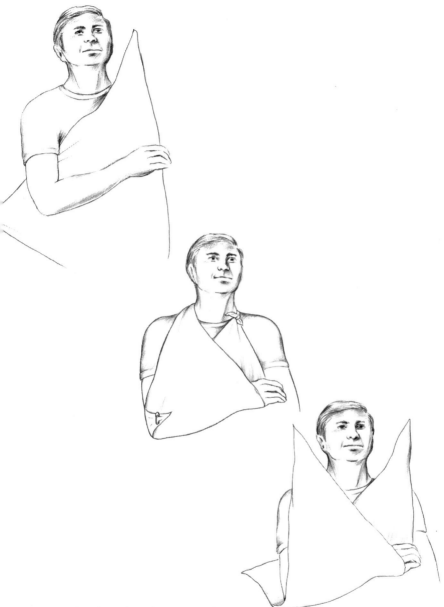

Figures 23 a, b, c. Step-by-step method of applying arm splint.

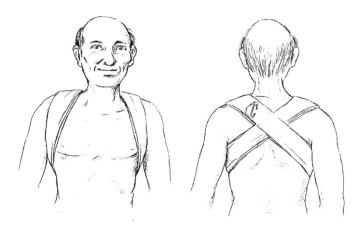

Figure 24. Figure-eight splint for fracture of collarbone.

shoulder a few times. The arm on the side of the fracture can be supported in a sling to help immobilize the injured part (see Fig. 24).

C. **Skull Injuries and Fractures** See Head Injuries, in chapter 3, page 35.

D. **Neck Injuries** The care needed in the management of an injured neck cannot be emphasized enough. If the victim complains in any way of a snapping or painful sensation in the neck, whether or not there are signs of weakness or paralysis of the extremities or numbness or loss of touch or pain sensation anywhere in the body, the patient should be treated as having a possible neck fracture.

What To Do

1. Wherever the patient is lying, either in the water or on the deck, he should be left and supported in that position until a board or door—large enough to maintain rigid alignment of the head and body—is brought.

2. A team should be assembled and coordinated efforts should be made to roll the patient over, slip the board under, and roll the patient back onto the board, at the same time supporting the head very carefully in line with the trunk. Maintain a slight traction stretching the neck during the procedure. This position with respect to alignment of the neck and the body should be maintained throughout this entire maneuver, much as one might roll a log from side to side.
3. The head must be taped and/or propped in place by appropriate padding or pillowing so that there is no tendency for the head to rotate or change position with respect to the body with any movement (see Fig. 25).
4. Medical attention should be sought immediately as this is a critical injury that does require careful transportation and medical management.

Method of immobilizing head and neck when possible neck fracture is suspected.

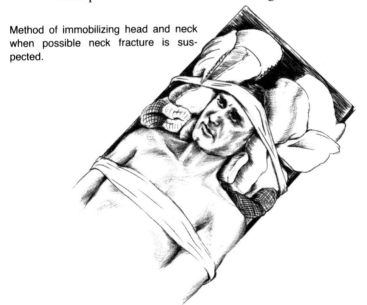

Figure 25. Immobilizing head and neck.

5. For pain, the patient may be given pain medication by mouth or by injection if available.
6. Paralyzed extremities must be carefully attended to and should not be permitted to get into uncomfortable or abnormal positions. The victim may not be able to move or to feel sensation in the extremity to warn of impending injury. Pad bony prominences, such as elbows and knees, that may be resting on hard surfaces.

E. Injuries of the Back Fractures or possible fractures of the back should be managed as described above for injuries of the neck, keeping the spine supported in a straight immobilized position and putting slight traction on the lower extremities. A board or door should be used to support and/or during transportation. Never place a victim with a possible back fracture in a hammock or on a soft stretcher.

Open Fracture

When there is a simple fracture, splinting and eventual setting by a physician are usually effective and readily accomplished. A much more serious injury has been incurred when the fracture has broken through the skin. It must be considered contaminated even though the wound may not appear grossly soiled.

What To Do
1. Attempt to reduce the bleeding by applying a pressure dressing (see page 13), taking care not to push dirt or bone fragments further into the wound.
2. Do not irrigate or wash, as this may further aggravate and contaminate deeper areas of the wound.
3. Do not attempt to realign the bone or allow the bone ends to withdraw underneath the skin or back through the wound, unless more than 5 hours will pass before professional help can be reached. If an extensive period of time is expected to pass before help can be reached, it is better to allow the bone

ends to be withdrawn into the wound, exerting steady, gentle traction on the extremity. This should be maintained during and after splinting.
4. If medical attention is delayed, penicillin, 2 tablets every four hours, should be given.
5. Apply a light dressing and attempt to fix the injured extremity in such a position as to immobilize it and keep it from further damage.
6. Get professional medical attention.

Fractures are painful, and moving the injured part hurts more. Both victim and first-aid attendant must be courageous. Pain medications such as Talwin® by mouth or injection are helpful. Proper splinting and immobilization will produce the most relief, and will be well worth the pain endured during the process.

Chapter 8

General Body Disorders: When Nothing Is Go

We have described a number of specific systems and regions of the body that might suffer from accidents or injuries, or that might need urgent care or treatment during a boating experience. In many instances certain injuries may cover more than one system or region, and wherever possible this has been referred to in more than one chapter.

It is well recognized, however, that there are some so-called generalized systemic reactions that involve the body as a whole and do not lend themselves well to a discussion of any specialized system or region—for example, seasickness and hangovers.

SEASICKNESS

One such condition, and perhaps the most common, is seasickness. There is probably no simple, single good treatment for this notorious malady, otherwise there would be no need for the volumes of rhetoric about it. This disorder usually results from a combined distortion between the senses, particularly between the eyes and the balancing mechanism in the inner ear. To this is added the complexity of psychogenic factors, aggravated by such items as lack of sleep or preexisting disorders. When this is further complicated by unpleasant sensations, such as odors often found below deck, there is hardly anyone who can resist such a barrage of discomforting stimuli, wrapped up in the rocking motion of the waves, and seasickness results.

What To Do
1. The best place to be is usually topside and midship where the actual motion is minimized both in pitch and roll directions.
2. There are always exceptions—some people feel much better lying in a bunk below deck.
3. At the first sign of seasickness, dry foods may be more helpful than a large quantity of liquids.
4. Getting busily preoccupied with some chores or duties may wipe out all the discomfort.
5. Antinausea or seasick pills may be taken. These pills must be individually tested to find out which works best for each person. They tend to work differently in different individuals.

    Many of the common seasickness pills on the drugstore shelf today are similar preparations under different brand names. Most can be chewed and then swallowed. The old Bucladin® was a particularly effective medication, but it was removed from the market by edict, because of concern for potential side effects, and replaced with a preparation similar to many others and somewhat less

effective than the original. Any of these preparations may be taken, one tablet every 4–6 hours, for prevention or treatment of seasickness.
6. If the situation has progressed beyond the pill-taking stage and nausea and vomiting preclude any oral intake of drugs, medication may be administered very effectively rectally, in the form of a suppository. Compazine®, 25 mg (adult dose), Dramamine®, or Phenergan®, 50 mg, in suppository form, can be inserted every 4–6 hours for intractable seasickness. After subsidence of symptoms, if there has been severe vomiting and dehydration, the victim should gradually rehydrate with a saline solution (one level teaspoonful of salt in a full 8-ounce glass of water) or salty liquids, such as tomato juice.
7. The best treatment for seasickness is always prevention: get plenty of rest, take prophylactic seasickness pills if you have a tendency to get seasick, stay out of odorous, closed areas such as the galley or below deck, and eat solid food regularly, or even small dry meals more frequently than usual. In addition, a well-directed prayer can do no harm.

HANGOVERS

Any book on first aid would certainly be incomplete without advice on a malaise commonly found on board ship, among other places: the hangover. Even though man has learned how to fly to the moon, there is still no single, simple, effective method for treating this particular misery, in spite of the fact that the problem has been around since man first learned how to mix up a brew.

We have learned, however, that the probabilities of the combination of dehydration and depletion of salt may be factors in this disorder. The following suggestions are therefore provided:

What To Do
1. Drink a salty solution such as salted tomato juice. This supplies the fluids, salt, and blood chemicals that may be depleted. (This may explain why morning-after Bloody Marys are reputed to be so helpful; the gin or vodka in a Bloody Mary does not necessarily offer any additional therapeutic effects.) In the absence of salty tomato juice, any other salty drink, or a level teaspoonful of salt in a full glass of ice-cold water may be sipped.
2. Two Tylenol® tabs may be given for headache.
3. Thiamine or Vitamin B_1, 50 mg tablet, may be taken and repeated in 2–4 hours.
4. For severe nausea, Compazine®, 10–20 mg or Phenergan®, 25–50 mg, may be taken by mouth or as rectal suppository every 4 hours if necessary. This may produce drowsiness.
5. If all else fails, sleep it off if your crew will let you.

EXPOSURE

Heat Exhaustion

Heat exhaustion is just what the name implies: marked exhaustion, weakness, appearance of shock, *low* body temperature, dryness or dehydration, and often muscle cramps, resulting from extensive exposure to heat with persistent loss of fluids through perspiration. Along with the perspiration goes salt, which, when deficient, also contributes to the symptoms of this disorder.

What To Do
1. Remove the person to the shade, but ice or strenuous cooling measures are not necessary.
2. Encourage drinking of salty fluids such as saline solution (one level teaspoonful salt to one full 8-ounce glass of water) or salty drinks, such as tomato

juice with added salt. This may be repeated in 15–30 minutes. Salt pills with water may be used instead.
3. Loosen the clothing so that air can circulate freely and perspiration evaporate.
4. If the patient is pale, weak, and faint, have him lie flat and elevate his legs.
5. If nausea and vomiting make it impossible to take fluids orally, the patient may require medical attention and intravenous fluids.

Heat Stroke

This is a most serious calamity, with a high rate of mortality, and must be vigorously treated. Heat stroke results from prolonged exposure to heat, ultimately causing a dysfunction of the body's heat-regulating mechanisms. The victim will be *hot* and dry instead of sweating and will be in a shocklike state, perhaps unconscious.

Elevated fever may vary as high as 106 degrees F. or more orally. This is a primary difference from the heat exhaustion described above. The following steps may be used in any case of elevated fever and should be vigorously applied depending on the severity of the problem.

What To Do

1. Remove the patient from exposure to heat and remove his clothes so that heat can radiate freely from the body.
2. Immerse patient in cool water or sponge off with cool water, mixed half and half with rubbing alcohol, or place a damp sheet over the patient and fan the sheet to evaporate the water and produce a cooling effect.
3. Keep a careful watch on the temperature to be sure it falls and, just as importantly, that it remains down and doesn't rise again when cooling measures have been discontinued. For particularly resistant high temperature, ice packs may be placed on the palm side of the wrists, in the armpits (axillae), and about

the ankles to cool the blood traversing the major blood vessels that are very near the skin in those areas.
4. Nothing should be given by mouth unless the patient is conscious and able to swallow, in which case give iced saline (one level teaspoon of salt in full glass of water).
5. The patient should be referred for medical attention as soon as possible.

Environmental Exposure

Exposure is a common term used in the newspapers to describe the condition of those lost in the wilderness or at sea over periods of days or longer. The effects of exposure will depend, in part, on the conditions to which the victim has been exposed. Exposure is almost always the effect of combined deficiency of food and water, low environmental temperatures, and energy loss from overexertion.

What To Do
1. The best treatment, as with nearly all first-aid insults, is prevention, through proper preparation with food and water, appropriate clothing, planning, and conservation of energy.
2. Rescue of one suffering from exposure requires careful restraint on the part of victim as well as rescuer. Moderation is the word, with gradual warming, drinking small quantities of liquids (non-alcoholic), and eating bland, soft, or liquid foods such as soups, stews, and soft, well-cooked meats, vegetables, and hot cereals.

UNCONSCIOUSNESS

Fainting

This is a frightening experience, more so for those in attendance than for the victim who, more often than not, does not have a serious disease or condition. As long as there is protection from injuries to himself or herself while falling, there will seldom be a serious outcome. But those in attendance will go through throes of anxiety and push the panic button unless they have some previously arranged plan of action.

Most fainting episodes are vaso-vagal syncope and are the result of a slowing of the pulse and dilation of abdominal blood vessels with resultant deficiency of pressure of blood from the heart up to the head. In some people this results from seeing blood, being stuck with a needle, sometimes from fright, after a heavy drinking and eating bout, or, occasionally, just from getting up from a lying position too rapidly.

In any of the above instances, consciousness readily returns as the victim assumes a horizontal position. This allows the blood to reach the head again.

What To Do

1. Protect the faint or fainting individual from falling with resultant injury.
2. Stretch the victim out flat or, if not totally unconscious and seated, have him or her lean forward in a seated position with the head lowered below the knees.
3. Loosen tight clothing.
4. With the victim lying flat, elevate the lower extremities.
5. Check the pulse either at the wrist or carotid areas just below the angle of the jaw, or by listening to the pulse by placing the ear directly on the anterior chest to the left of the breastbone. This is to confirm that there is a slow and regular pulse, and thus rule out fainting or unconsciousness due to a disturbance of the heart rhythm.
6. Inhaling spirits of ammonia may be helpful.
7. After regaining consciousness, the patient should be allowed to rest until stable and should get up very slowly and assure steadiness before walking.

GENERAL BODY DISORDERS 97

8. The victim should be observed carefully for 12–24 hours and should refrain from assuming any responsibilities or positions or stations wherein recurrent symptoms could result in injury to himself or others

Unconsciousness with Convulsions

The most common example of this disorder is epilepsy, in which case there is usually a prior history of similar episodes. Here again the prime effort of those in attendance is to protect the victim from self-injury. This consists essentially of patiently biding time until the episode ends—which it will almost invariably do spontaneously.

What To Do

1. Protect the victim from falling and injuring himself or herself.
2. If possible place a soft object between the teeth, preferably padded, so that the tongue will not get caught between clenched teeth. A thick piece of rubber, a loop of half-inch or thicker line, a padded stick, or the end of a leather knife sheath are examples of handy items that might be available for such an emergency. Do not attempt to pry open the victim's mouth if the teeth are already clenched and the tongue is not caught.
3. Loosen clothing.
4. In case the patient is thrashing or moving so as to possibly injure any part of his anatomy, rather than restrain the individual, place padding in appropriate areas to protect him or her from injury. These episodes are usually self-limiting and the patient will gradually relax and regain consciousness with some residual but temporary confusion and a headache, but generally with no serious ill effects if this is a typical epileptic seizure.
5. During the course of the episode, there may be loss of sphincter control of urine or bowels.

6. Most important is reassurance of the patient and all those in attendance.

Faintness and Unconsciousness Due to Heart Irregularity

The description of cardiac arrest or sudden cessation of heartbeat was discussed under Closed-Chest Resuscitation in chapter 1, page 8 and chapter 4 under Cardiac Arrest, page 57. Of course, with complete cessation of the heartbeat, a critical situation exists and must be treated with the ABCs described in those chapters.

If there is the possibility of an irregularity, listen to the chest over the heart area to the left of the breastbone with the ear directly on the chest wall, or feel for pulses at the wrists (see Fig. 2) or carotid areas just below the angle of the jaw on either side of the neck (see Fig. 3). It may be reassuring that a pulse is found, but it may be rapid or irregular. In such a case the breathing may be continuing at a normal or somewhat rapid rate, the color may remain good, and the patient may not completely lose consciousness but become only faint or woozy.

What To Do

1. Lay the patient down on a firm surface, protecting him or her from injury.
2. Loosen all clothing.
3. Elevate the lower extremities.
4. Locate the carotid pulse just below the angle of the jaw on either side of the neck (see Fig. 3) and gently but firmly massage the neck over this pulse, one side at a time, while the patient is lying flat. While doing this, one should feel or listen for the pulse over the heart to see if there is any change in the rate or rhythm. The pulse may suddenly slow to half, or a third, or a fourth of its previous rhythm, or there may be a return to a perfectly normal basic rhythm. If this fails to result from massage on one side, try the other side. **WARNING:** Do not massage both sides of the neck simultaneously, especially in an elderly patient.

5. If this fails, have the patient blow against a closed tube while holding the nose and release the closed tube suddenly so as to relieve the pressure of the chest rapidly.
6. In any case of heart arrhythmia, unless the patient has previously had similar experiences, and appropriate medical advice and medication with instructions are readily available, this problem should be referred to a medical doctor. If at any time during efforts to assist such a patient the breathing or heartbeat stops and the patient convulses, proceed as in Cardiac Arrest, page 57.

PROGRESSIVE CONFUSION AND LETHARGY OR DROWSINESS

Confusion and drowsiness may represent a serious brain injury due to a number of conditions related to the circulation or injury of the brain. (See Head Injuries, chapter 2, page 35.)

Diabetes

Diabetes may be suspected in anyone who suddenly becomes confused, lethargic, or drowsy. If an individual has been nauseated, vomiting, feverish, urinating excessively, or has omitted taking insulin or antidiabetic medications, one may suspect a developing diabetic coma. The patient may complain of severe thirst, hunger, and feel and look very dehydrated. Marked weakness will be noted. If the patient has any methods for testing urine, it will usually show positive for sugar. In such case, the patient should be urged to take additional insulin immediately and medical attention be sought regarding further management.

What To Do

1. A glass of saline solution (one level teaspoonful of salt in a full 8-ounce glass of water) may be given and repeated at half-hour intervals as long as the patient is not nauseated or vomiting.

2. Further management will depend on the response of the patient; it may take the form of repeated doses of insulin and continued administration of saline solution. This may, in part, be guided by repeated urine tests for sugar and acetone if these tests are available and, if possible, should be under the direction of a physician and in the hospital.

Insulin Reaction

Insulin reaction or shock is the opposite effect of diabetic coma. In this case there also may be mental confusion and eventual loss of consciousness. The patient, however, is apt to be very nervous, agitated, warm, and perspiring, with a rapid pulse. There may be a decrease in urination and, on questioning, the patient may recall having taken insulin or diabetic medications by mouth without having eaten an adequate amount of food. Another possibility is that the individual may have become seasick and vomited his food so that he has a relative deficiency of sugar in relation to the insulin in his system.

What To Do

1. Encourage the patient to drink orange juice, sugar water, or eat candy or sugar cubes. Do not encourage any oral intake if the patient is unconscious or unable to swallow. In such circumstances seek medical help as soon as possible.
2. If the patient is confused, he or she may have to be cajoled, urged, and even fooled into taking the sugar by mouth. This may become a game of wits between patient and would-be rescuers.
3. If in doubt as to whether a diabetic patient is having symptoms of coma with *too little* insulin and too much blood sugar, or insulin reaction due to *too much* insulin and too little sugar, favor the insulin-reaction probability and give the patient immediate calories in the form of some sugar-containing preparation such as candy, orange juice, or sugar.

4. If the patient gradually clears mentally, sits up, looks around, and asks what has been going on, one may be temporarily reassured, but be careful and forewarned that if the patient has taken a long-acting antidiabetic medication, he or she could slip back into insulin shock within 30 minutes to an hour after the present supply of sugar has been metabolized. One should, therefore, feed the individual with some more solid foods such as milk, meat, or eggs containing protein and then continue subsequent meals at appropriate intervals, watching carefully for 12–24 hours for signs of recurrence.

Chapter 9

Water Safety

For information that may save your life or the life of a loved one, all boaters should have the American National Red Cross book, *Life Saving, Rescue, and Water Safety*, which has much to teach anyone in or around the water. Some rules of water safety bear repetition at this time with the understanding that any simple and limited list such as this leaves much unsaid.

BE PREPARED
1. Learn to swim if you are going to be in or about the water and, especially, out on boats.
2. When swimming, always use the buddy system even in a private pool at home.

3. Do not overestimate your ability, and do not leave an overturned boat in an effort to swim to a distant shore. Stay with your boat.
4. Do not swim immediately after eating or when severely overheated.
5. Be sure water is of adequate depth before diving.
6. Be aware of the possibility of sunburn even while swimming or snorkling. A smart swimmer without an adequate suntan or protective lotion will use a tee shirt and socks to cover exposed parts of the body, especially while snorkling.
7. Never swim in water when there is a threat of an electrical storm.
8. Never stand in water, especially barefoot, when using electrical tools. Always be sure electrical tools are grounded when around water or moisture.
9. A boat skipper or owner would be wise to have his life-saving credentials. The American National Red Cross offers courses of instruction and certification.
10. When throwing a flotation object tied to a line toward a swimmer, always throw the flotation object beyond the swimmer and draw it back toward him as you pull in the line.
11. Learn floating techniques, including how to inflate clothing to assist with flotation. This can be done by fanning air under a jacket or shirt tied or tightly fastened at the neck and open at the waist. A pair of trousers can also serve as a substitute life preserver by removing them and tying the ends of the legs together, then inflating the trousers with air held in by tightening the waist with the belt. The inflated legs may then be placed over the head much like a standard life preserver (see Fig. 26).
12. In extremely cold water keep clothes on as a means of retaining some heat. Don't swim to keep warm but rather simply stay afloat, conserving your energy as much as possible. Stay with your boat, and remember that the shore looks closer than it actually is.

DROWNING

In cases of drowning, begin artificial respiration as soon as possible. Do not waste time worrying about water in the lungs or loosening clothing. Do not turn the victim over on his stomach. Proceed with the ABCs (pages 8 and 57) without taking any time over preliminaries.

Immediate Steps

What To Do

1. Place the victim on his back.
2. Clear the mouth and throat of any obstructions to breathing.
3. Start mouth-to-mouth resuscitation.* If the stomach bulges, exert a moderate amount of pressure during expiration to rid the stomach of water and air. Pull victim on side to allow water to drain.
4. Check for heartbeat and pulse. If they are absent, start closed-chest compression (page 8).
5. Once the victim begins breathing, mouth-to-mouth respiration may be continued if natural breathing is shallow. Do not interfere with natural breath.
6. Watch for vomiting. If victim vomits while unconscious, turn him on the side to keep vomitus from entering the lungs.
7. Treat for shock (see page 14).

After Six to Twelve Hours

Keep the patient warm (but not hot) and comfortable. Elevate the lower part of the body. Give fluids in small amounts, such as warm water, tea, broth, or coffee. Give no alcoholic beverages.

---

*Artificial respiration using chest-pressure methods as were taught a few years ago are much less effective than mouth-to-mouth resuscitation techniques and have not been included in this book.

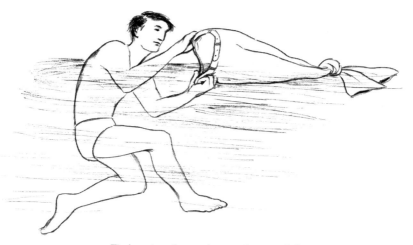

Tie legs together and scoop trousers full of air. Slip loop of legs over head and hold waist closed.

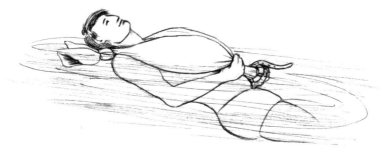

Figure 26. Impromptu life preserver.

Chapter 10

Your First-Aid Kit

What should be included in a first-aid kit?

There are probably as many answers to this question as there are people who have asked it. Throughout this book I have mentioned various drugs, supplies, instruments, and aids. Their uses and applications have been described as we went along.

I would like now to compile this list for you and briefly indicate their use. Wherever practical, I will refer to the descriptions in the text and the chart on page 6.

These are my personal choices as of this moment; they will undoubtedly change as new drugs and instruments appear on the market. In many cases, the names mentioned represent only one of a number of similar preparations that could be used interchangeably. There are certainly other choices that competent physicians might prefer over those mentioned in this book and, in all probability, I would have no argument with them. We all have our favorites and on any one occasion one drug may work better than another only to be reversed in efficiency on the next similar occasion.

One word of warning. Almost all drugs have potential side effects. Many are unpredictable. Some may be expected to be dangerous for certain people and contraindicated for those with certain preexisting conditions. Your own doctor should be consulted regarding your use of the preparations suggested here. You may have to request that he provide prescriptions for some of the preparations suggested. If symptoms persist, seek medical attention. Children should take one-third to one-half the adult dose—roughly proportionate to the weight of the child as compared to a 150-pound adult.

FOR INFECTIONS WITH FEVER

Antibiotics

Antibiotics should not be necessary and may not even be advisable in ordinary kits for short trips. When need is suspected, a doctor's opinion is advised. For longer trips, or whenever medical assistance may not be available for days, the following drugs may be useful:
1. Tetracycline (250 mg)—especially for bladder infections and when an allergy to pencillin is present, and for infections when penicillin is ineffective after 2 days. Two tablets or capsules, 4 times a day.
2. Penicillin (500 mg)—for infections with fever from other than bladder infections or if tetracycline is ineffective in 2 days. One tablet 4 times a day or every 4 hours.
3. Antibiotic ointments—for skin infections.
    a. Polysporin® is a general all-purpose skin antibiotic ointment. Apply twice a day.
    b. Mycolog® is an antibiotic ointment for fungus infections of the skin. Apply twice a day.

Note: Once started, these drugs should be continued for 7–10 days even though symptoms disappear, unless untoward reaction to the drug develops, such as rash or severe stomach upset.

FOR ALLERGIES

Antiallergy Drugs

1. Adrenalin® (epinephrine): injection (dilution 1–1000) 1 cc ampule should be available as emergency drug for acute anaphylactic (allergic) reaction or intractable asthma. This can be provided in disposable syringe with needle (see method of injection on page 49).*
2. Benadryl® (25 mg): one capsule for children or sensitive individuals, or 2 capsules—the usual adult dose—for allergic reaction as well as for sedation.
3. Chlortrimeton®: 8 mg, or 12 mg repetabs may be taken every 8–12 hours for longer action and somewhat less sedation.
4. Actifed® for nasal decongestion or allergy or for head-cold symptoms: one tablet every 8 hours.

*Remember, when injecting adrenalin using technique described, insert needle approximately halfway into the skin and inject one-half of the solution at a time, allowing 10–15 minutes to observe for effects. The remaining half of the contents of the syringe can then be injected if necessary.

FOR ASTHMA: BRONCHODILATORS

1. Theolair®: one tablet (250 mg) every 4–6 hours as necessary.
2. Bronkometer®: a last resort used as infrequently as possible.

FOR DIGESTIVE DISORDERS

Constipation

1. Milk of Magnesia: one or 2 tablespoonsful or 4–6 tablets as directed on the label.

2. Senokot®: 2 tablets or one teaspoonful of granules, once or twice daily as directed.
3. Dulcolax® suppository: insert rectally for effect in 15–30 minutes.
4. Fleet Phosphosoda®: 2–4 teaspoonsful as directed on label.
5. Fleet® enema: insert rectally for rapid (5-minute) and predictable effect.

Diarrhea
1. Lomotil® (on prescription): 1 or 2 tablets every 4 hours as necessary.
2. Kaopectate or Pepto-Bismol®: 2 tablespoonsful every 2 hours for four to six doses.
3. Neotracina® (over-the-counter in Mexico; not available in U.S.): may be taken 2 or 3 times a day as a prophylaxis against *"turista."* Check with your doctor first regarding contraindications.

Indigestion
1. Mylanta II®—or others, e.g., Maalox, Gelusil, etc.: 2 tablets one to 2 hours after meals and at bedtime or, as liquid, one or 2 tablespoonsful on similar schedule.
2. Charcodote®: 15 gm activated charcoal, for gaseous distress (with meals, and may also be used for swallowed poisons; see chapter 5, page 64).

FOR RESPIRATORY AILMENTS

Cough Suppressants
1. Robitussin DM®: for an adult, 1 tablespoonful every 3–4 hours.
2. Elixir Terpin Hydrate with codeine: one or 2 teaspoonsful every 3–4 hours for more potent cough suppression.
3. Saturated solution of potassium iodide (expectorant): 10 drops in water or juice every 4 hours.

Nasal or Sinus Blockage

Warning: Any nose drops or spray may be injurious when used too long. A course of 2 or 3 days followed by one or 2 days without use is urged.

1. Afrin®: spray every 12 hours as directed on container.
2. Sudafed® (nasal decongestant without antihistamine): one tablet 3–4 times a day.
3. Actifed® (nasal decongestant with antihistamine): one tablet every 8 hours for head cold or allergy.

FOR PAIN

Analgesics

1. Aspirin: 2 tablets every 4 hours with full 8-ounce glass of water for ordinary aches and pains and fever.
2. Tylenol®: 2 tablets every 4 hours with full 8-ounce glass of water—instead of aspirin may prevent stomach upset, or if patient takes anticoagulant (blood thinning) pills and should not take aspirin.
3. Tylenol® with 0.5 grain of codeine for more severe pain (one or 2 tablets every 3–4 hours). Empirin with 0.5 grain of codeine may be substituted.

Chest Pains

1. Nitroglycerine: one tablet under tongue for chest pain; repeat at 3- to 5-minute intervals if necessary, for three doses. If no relief, give Talwin®.
2. Talwin®, available on prescription only, as 50 mg tablets, or 30 mg ampules for injection: give one tablet every 4 hours for severe pain. For emergency treatment for severe pain if victim is unable to take medicine by mouth, inject one ampule (30 mg). See page 49 for method of injecting.

FOR SEASICKNESS

1. Bonine® or Antivert®, Bucladin®, Dramamine®: one tablet every 4–6 hours may be tried.
2. Phenergan®: 25–50 mg (50 mg adult dose). Or Compazine®: 5–25 mg (25 mg adult dose). Suppositories for more intractable vomiting—on prescription only.

FOR STINGS—INSECT OR SEA LIFE (NONPOISONOUS)

1. Adolph's Meat Tenderizer poultice for stings—except for wasps'.
2. Sodium bicarbonate poultice for all stings.
3. Either should be applied as a small mound of moistened powder (poultices) on wound site after thorough cleansing of wound.

FOR SUNBURN

1. White vinegar. Dilute one part to 3 of water for unbroken skin.

FOR SUNSCREEN

1. Maxifil®.
2. PreSun®.
3. Many similar alternative preparations.

FOR ACUTE ANXIETY AND INSOMNIA

1. Valium®: one or two 5 mg tablets every 4 hours or at bedtime.
2. Librium®: one or two 10 mg capsules, as recommended for Valium.

MISCELLANEOUS

1. Ace Bandage®: 3-inch width for sprains and dressings.

2. Adhesive tape: one- and 3-inch widths.
3. Airway (Resusitube®): to maintain open airway through mouth and for mouth-to-mouth breathing.
4. Band-Aids®: various sizes.
5. Betadine®: scrubbing antiseptic.
6. Valisone® ointment (or other similar steroid preparation): for skin irritation, itch, or superficial burn.
7. Gauze: sterile pads (3" x 3"), preferably Telfa® (nonadherent).
8. Hydrogen peroxide (3 percent solution): to irrigate wounds or obstructed ear canals.
9. Inflatable splints.
10. Kling®: self-adherent bandage dressing.
11. Lip pomade.
12. Newspaper rolls: can be used as splints for fractures of small bones.
13. Sanitary napkins (can also be used for pressure dressings).
14. Soap for salt water as well as fresh water.
15. Two sterile 2.5 cc disposable syringes with ¾" No. 25 needles on each syringe.
16. Steri-Strips®: sterile adhesive strips to close wound, instead of suture (see page 23).
17. Thermometer.
18. Lasix®, 40 mg, diuretic or water pill.

It is my fervent hope that you never need to use any of the advice or preparations suggested in this book. Just having them near may make your trip a little more comfortable, and a lot safer, for you and your crew.

Smooth sailing, and a safe return!

Index

Numbers in italics refer to illustrations.

ABCs, 8–12, 57–59, 105
Abdominal pain, acute, 69–75
  appendicitis, 71
  checklist for, 74–75
  gallbladder disease, 70–71
  gas pocket, 73–74
  kidney stone, 72–73
  location of organs, *70*
  mittelschmerz, 70–71
  muscle strain, 73
  pancreatitis, 72
  See also Peptic ulcer
Abrasions, 18–19
Abscesses, 28–30
Acute anxiety, first aid for, 111
Adhesive tape, applying to chest wall, *52*
Airway. *See* ABCs
Allergies, 47–51
  anaphylactic shock, 51
  asthma, 47–49
  first aid for, 108
  injection procedure, 49–50
American National Red Cross, 102
Analgesics (pain killers), 6, 110
Anaphylactic shock, 51
Angina pectoris, 55–56
Antacids, 66
Antiallergy drugs, 6, 108
Antibiotics, 6, 107–8
  ointments, 6, 107
Antihistamines, 6
Antiseptics, 6
Appendicitis, 71
Appendix, *70*
Arm, control of bleeding in, *20*
Arm splint, applying, *85*
Artery:
  bleeding, 14
  pulse, 10–12
Artificial respiration, 105
Asthma attacks, 47–49
  first aid for, 108
Athlete's foot, 30

Avulsion, 19–20

Back injuries (or possible fractures), 88
Barbs, puncture wounds from, 26–27
Bee stings, 24
Black eye, 39–40
Black widow spider, *25*, 26
Bladder infection, 77
Bleeding, control of, 14
  in arm, *20*
  pressure points for palpating pulses and
    compressing arteries for, *21*
  tourniquet for, *22*
Blindness, sun or snow, 40
Blocked nose, 43
Boating injuries:
  breathing and heartbeat, 47–61
  crisis, rescue, and treatment, 4–16
  first-aid kit, 106–112
  gastrointestinal tract, 62–75
  general body disorders, 90–101
  genitourinary system, 76–78
  head, 35–46
  introduction to, 1–3
  musculoskeletal, 79–89
  skin, 17–34
  water safety, 102–5
Boils and abscesses, 28–30
Breathing, obstructed, 45–46
Breathing and heartbeat, 47–61
  allergies, 47–51
  carbon monoxide poisoning, 54
  after cardiac arrest, reestablishing,
    58–59
  chest injuries, 51–53
  drowning, 61
  heart injury, 55–61
  hyperventilation, 53–54
  mouth-to-mouth, *9*
  pleurisy-pneumonia, 54–55
  See also ABCs
Broken nose, 42
Bronchodilators, 6, 108

INDEX

Bruised eye, 39–40
Burns, 30–33
    assessing percentage of, *31*

Carbon monoxide poisoning, 54
Cardiac arrest, 57–59
Carotid artery location (to feel for pulsations with heartbeat), *12*
Cathartics, 7
Chapped lips, 43–44
Chemical burns, 33
Chest compression, *13*
Chest injuries, 51–53
Chest pains, first aid for, 110
Chest wall, applying adhesive tape to, *52*
Choking, 45–46
Circulation, after cardiac arrest, re-establishing, 59
    See also ABCs
Closed chest compression, *13*
Closed (simple) fractures, 83–88
Collarbone fracture, 84–86
    figure-eight splint, *86*
Confusion and lethargy, 99-101
Conjunctivitis (infected conjunctiva), 38
Consciousness, head injury, 35–37
Constipation, 68–69
    first aid for, 108–9
Constricted pupil, *36*
Contaminated food poisoning, 64–65
Convulsions, unconsciousness with, 97–98
Coral snakes, 24–25
    puncture wounds from, 26–27
Cough suppressants, 6, 109
CPR (cardio-pulmonary resuscitation), 8–12
Crisis, rescue, and treatment, 4–16
    ABCs, 8–12
    bleeding, 14
    carotid artery location, *12*
    checklist for, 16
    chest compression, *13*
    equipment available and, 5–8
    medication, 6–8
    mouth-to-mouth breathing, *9*
    pulse location, *11*
    rescue situation, 5
    resuscitation of an infant, *15*
    shock, 14–16
    when victim is unconscious, 8–14

Deafness, sudden, 41
Dental problems, 44
Diabetic coma, 100
Diarrhea, 7, 69
    first aid for, 109
Digestive aids, 7

Digestive disorders, 65–69
    acute abdominal pain, 69–75
    constipation, 68–69
    diarrhea, 69
    first aid for, 108–9
    gastroenteritis, 67–68
    indigestion, 65–66
    peptic ulcers, 66–67
Dilated pupil, *36*
Dislocations (bones out of joint), 81
Dizziness, 41–42
Drowning or near-drowning, 61, 105
    after 6 to 12 hours (what to do), 105
    immediate steps, 105
Drowsiness, 99–101
Duodenal ulcers, 66–67

Earache (otalgia), 40–41
Ears, 40–42
    decreased hearing, 41
    dizziness, 41–42
Electrical grounding, 103
Enema, 69
Environmental exposure, 95
Epididymis, 78
Epilepsy, 97–98
Esophagitis, 66
Exposure, 93–95
Extremities, fractures, 83–84
Eyes, 38–40
    bruised or black eye, 39–40
    foreign body in, 38, *39*
    irrigating, *33*
    pinkeye, 38
    snow or sun blindness, 40

Fainting, 95–97
Faintness and unconsciousness, due to heart irregularity, 98–99
Fever, 6
Figure-eight splint, *86*
First-aid kit, 106–12
    for actue anxiety and insomnia, 111
    for allergies, 108
    for asthma, 108
    for digestive disorders, 108–9
    for infections and fever, 107–8
    miscellaneous, 111–12
    for pain, 110
    for respiratory ailments, 109–10
    for seasickness, 111
    for stings, 111
    for sunburn, 111
    for sunscreen, 111
First-degree burns, 32
    characteristics of, 30

Fish, poisonous, 26, 27
　puncture wounds from, 26–27
Fish poisoning, 65
Fishhook in skin, *27–28*
Food, dislodging from windpipe, 45–46, *46*
Forearm, splinting fracture of, *83*
Fractured ribs, 51–52
Fractures, 81–89
　general measures for, 81–82
　open, 88–89
　splinting, *83, 85, 86*
Fresh water, near-drowning in, 61
Frostbite, 34
Fungus infection, 6

Gallbladder, *70*
Gallbladder disease, acute, 70–71
Gas pocket, 73–74
Gastroenteritis (the "GIs"), 67–68
Gastrointestinal tract, 62–75
　acute abdominal pain, 69–75
　digestive disorders, 65–69
　poisoning, 62–65
General body disorders, 90–101
　confusion and lethargy, 99–101
　exposure, 93–95
　hangovers, 97–98
　seasickness, 91–92
　unconsciousness, 95–99
Genitourinary system, 76–78

Hangovers, 97–98
"Hardened artery," 56
Head injuries, 35–46
　conscious and unconscious, 35–37
　ears, 40–42
　eyes, 38–40
　mouth, 43–46
　nose, 42–43
Hearing, sudden decrease in, 41
Heart attack, 56–57
Heart failure, 60–61
Heart injury, 55–61
　angina pectoris, 55–56
　cardiac arrest, 57–59
　near-drowning, 61
　See also ABCs; Breathing and heartbeat
Heart irregularity, fainting and unconsciousness, 98–99
Heart sounds, area to listen for, *58*
Heartbeat. *See* Breathing and heartbeat
Heat exhaustion, 93–94
Heat stroke, 94–95
Heimlich maneuver, 45, *46*
Hyperventilation, 53–54

Incisions and lacerations, 20–23
Indigestion, 65–66
　first aid for, 109
Infant, resuscitation of, *15*
Infections with fever, first aid for, 107–8
Injection procedure, 49–50, *50*
Insect wounds, poisonous, 26
Insomnia, first aid for, 111
Instruments, sterilizing, 30
Insulin reaction, 100–101
Intestinal spasm, 73
Intramuscular injection, sites for, *50*
Irrigating the eye, *33*

Joint sprains, 80–81

Kidney, *70*
Kidney stone, passing, 72–73

Lacerations, 20–23
Large intestines, *70*
Life preserver, impromptu, *104*
Life Saving, Rescue, and Water Safety
　(American National Red Cross), 102
Ligaments, 80
Lips, chapped or sunburned, 43–44
Lymph glands, 45

Marine life, injury by, 26–27
Medication, 6–8
Mittelschmerz, 70–71
Molluscs, puncture wounds from, 26–27
Mouth, 43–46
　chapped and sunburned lips, 43–44
　dental problems, 44
　obstructed breathing, 45–46
　sore throat, 44–45
Mouth-to-mouth breathing, *9*
Muscle injury, spasm and swelling, 80
Muscle strain, acute, 73
Musculoskeletal injuries, 79–89
　dislocations, 81
　fractures, 81–89
　joint sprains, 80–81
　muscle injury, 80

Nasal blockage, first aid for, 110
Nasal decongestant, 7
Nausea control, 7
Near-drowning, 61
Neck, method of immobilizing head and, *87*
Neck injuries, 86–88
Normal pupil, *36*

INDEX

Nose, 42–43
  broken, 42
  stuffy or blocked, 43
Nosebleeds, 42

Obstructed breathing, 45–46
Open fracture, 88–89
Organs, location of, *70*
Ovaries, *70*

Pain, first aid for, 110
Pancreas, *70*
Pancreatitis, acute, 72
Panic, avoiding, 5
Penetrating chest wound, 52–53
Peptic ulcers, 66–67
Pinkeye, 38
Pleurisy-pneumonia, 54–55
Poisoning, 62–65
  carbon monoxide, 54
  contaminated food, 64–65
  ingestion of toxic fish, 65
  insect wounds, 26
  by toxic material, 62–64
Poisonous snakes, 24–25
Poultice, 24
Pulse, location, *11*
Puncture wounds, 23–28
Pupil reactions, *36*

Reproductive system, problems of, 78
Respiratory ailments, first aid for, 109–10
Resuscitation of an infant, *15*

Salt water, near-drowning in, 61
Scorpion, *25*, 26
Scrotum, injury or infection of, 78
Sea snake bites, 24–25
Sea urchin, wound from barb, 27
Seasickness, 91–92
  first aid for, 111
Secondary shock, 15–16
Second-degree burns, 32
  characteristics of, 30
Shock, 12–16
Sinus blockage, first aid for, 110
Skin, 17–34
  boils and abscesses, 28–30
  burns, 30–33
  frostbite, 34
  wounds, 18–28
Skull injuries and fractures. *See* Head injuries
Snakebites, 24–25
Snow or sun blindness, 40
Sore throat, 44–45
Spiders, poisonous:
  black widow, *25*, 26
  violin (brown recluse), *25*, 26
Spines, puncture wounds from, 26–27
Splinting for forearm, *83*
Sprains, joint, 80–81
Stings, 7
  first aid for, 111
Stomach, *70*
  acid, 65–66
  gas, 65–66
  ulcers, 66–67
Stuffy nose, 43
Sun blindness, 40
Sunburn, first aid for, 111
Sunburn and sunscreen lotions, 7
Sunburned lips, 43–44
Sunscreen, first aid for, 111

Tails, puncture wounds from, 26–27
Third-degree burns, 32–33
  characteristics of, 30–31
Throat, sore, 44–45
Toothache, 44
Tourniquet, how to apply, *22*
Toxic fish poisoning, 65
Toxic material, poisoning by, 62–64
Tranquilizers, 7

Ulcers, 66–67
  ruptured, 67
Unconsciousness, 95–99
  ABCs for, 8–12
  with convulsions, 97–98
  fainting, 95–97
  heart irregularity, 98–99
  See also Head injuries
Unequal pupil sizes, *36*
Urinary retention, 76–77
Urinary system, problems of. 76–78

Vaginal bleeding, excessive, 78
Venomous snakes, 24–25

Wasp stings, 24
Water safety, 102–5
  being prepared, 102–3
  drowning, 105
  impromptu life preserver, *104*
Windpipe, food blockage, how to dislodge, 45–46, *46*
Wounds, 18–28
  abrasions, 18–19
  avulsion, 19–20
  chest wall, 52–53
  incisions and lacerations, 20–23
  puncture, 23–28